Bedtime Stories for Stressed Adults

Deep Sleep Stories to Reduce Stress, Anxiety, and Insomnia

David Grifone

Table of Contents

Introduction

Mindfulness meditation is the kind of meditation we will be getting into. You may have a certain impression of mindfulness because of how popular it has become in public conversation. As I'm about to show you, mindfulness isn't only a good way to reduce stress but an ancient practice that will transport you into a deeper level of consciousness.

This level of consciousness is known as the unconscious. As you may have known already, this is the part of your mind where your dreams take place. It's no wonder that learning how to sleep and learning mindfulness meditation are so connected; for both of them, we have to communicate with our unconscious minds. That means learning this practice doesn't just serve as a tool for getting to bed at a decent hour. Mindfulness will make you wiser and even calmer during the day when you aren't trying to sleep.

Now, meditation is a rich subject that authors have written thousands of books about. We don't have the space to cover everything about it here. That doesn't mean you won't learn a lot, though. In just a page, I can tell you all you need to know to meditate correctly. It is a practice that goes perfectly with reading bedtime stories. Both will help you sleep.

Stories and meditations have a lot in common, too. I want to give you some exposition for what mindfulness meditation is all about. We'll also be making connections between mindfulness meditation, storytelling, and sleep.

What is mindfulness? You may still have this question, and I have a direct answer for you that is surprisingly hard to find elsewhere. In short, mindfulness is noticing what is there.

When you are mindful, you pay attention. Getting a handle on what mindfulness is may require considering the opposite of mindfulness. Think about the difference between focus and distraction. When you have a big project at home or at work, they are the two things you tend to switch between.

It's strange because we like to convince ourselves that we are always making progress on the task, but the truth is, either you are focused on the task and work on it, or you are not. That is, either you are mindful of the task and actively making progress on it, or you are distracted and not working on it at all.

Everyone struggles with this. It is simply a part of the human experience to go between focus and distraction. It makes sense for there are various sensory stimuli for us to lose ourselves in.

It doesn't necessarily mean we have to surrender to it. Mindfulness helps you notice what is happening. When you notice what is actually going on in your mind and in the world around you, you will be left with no choice but to accept the fact

5

that you are distracted — that you aren't doing the task you set out to do.

We can come to this conclusion without mindfulness, but it is much harder because the sensory stimuli draw us in so well that we don't even get a chance to evaluate what we are doing.

Take a moment to consider how this connects with reading stories. When you listen to a story, you have to focus on it to get anything out of it. This is what makes narrated stories so special compared to the ones we watch on the screen. We don't have to be especially mindful when the story is being told to us with a visual medium. It gives everything to you on a silver platter.

With sleep, we have to be mindful, so we can pay attention to just one thing and let our minds wander with it until our unconscious takes over our conscious mind. The key to sleeping with mindfulness is that the object of our attention needs to be fictional, so we use our unconscious instead of our conscious. This is where stories come in.

The current science on the human brain backs up the idea that engaging the unconscious will help us sleep. Just like meditation, neuroscience (the science of the brain) is an expansive topic, so we will only do a brief run-down here.

But in few words, the way scientists now understand the brain is through the paradigm of neural networks. You can think of neural networks as wires on a circuit board. If you're not a computer person, you can think of neural networks as constellations. The stars are your neurons (brain cells), and the lines connecting the constellations are your synaptic connections, which are the links between your neurons.

Then we have the neural networks or the constellations in this analogy. Your brain has many neural networks, but there are a few main ones that we will talk about here. You already know the idea of the left brain and right brain, and that idea is relatively solid.

But your neural networks are much more useful for understanding the human brain because they connect all the neurons in your brain to one another. The two neural networks we are concerned with are called the default mode network and the executive functioning network.

The executive functioning network is the neural network; we do not want to engage this when reading stories or getting to sleep. When we engage this network, we are too focused on what is going on in front of us to get our unconscious mind active. The executive functioning network is the neural network we use to brush our hair, ride a motorcycle, and admire art. It is the network we use to do things in the here and now.

Then we have the default mode network. This is the neural network we use to think about the past and future. We use it to imagine things that are not there, for we use it to see the story scenes the author is trying to paint. As you might imagine, the default mode network is the network you need to engage in order to tap into your unconscious and get to sleep.

Now that you have a scientific understanding of mindfulness in plain English — which is hard to find these days — you know how you can get your mind off of your daily struggles and into the unconscious world of sleep and dreams. You know everything you need to know to start meditating.

The first thing you do in mindfulness meditation is focusing on your breath. People teaching newcomers how to do this tend to overemphasize how you sit, where your hands go, and small things like this. Don't worry about these things; all you need to do is get into a comfortable position that you won't keep changing in and out of. From there, you start breathing deeply and focus on your breath.

Mindfulness meditation is easy to understand but hard to do, so I don't need to give you more instructions. All I can give you from here is some advice.

For starters, leave behind all the prior conceptions you had about meditation. None of that matters anymore.

You might have heard already that you should "clear your mind." This may be something that you can accomplish with mindfulness meditation; it's true. But seeing this as the goal this early on is detrimental to successful meditation. This early on in your mindfulness meditation practice, you are extremely unlikely to reach a state of tranquility that could qualify as clearing your mind. An active attempt to reach this state will just keep you from doing the most basic thing in meditation, so don't worry about it right now. It is something you will be able to achieve later on, but not if you keep getting frustrated by not clearing your mind.

That leads us to the next piece of advice. Many newcomers to mindfulness meditation give up on it early on because they have heard other people tell them what a unique, mind-altering experience they had when meditating, then they try to meditate, and nothing like this happens.

They are faced with their own breathing and the thoughts that flow through their brain instead of any sort of life-changing experience. You can't let yourself give up the possibility of that experience by giving up because you don't get it right away. You could meditate for a year before you get that experience. But if you actually meditate every day and you don't stop, your mind will be cleared, and you will have that experience one day. Be patient with it, and it will come.

I have one last piece of advice on mindfulness meditation before we move on to the stories. Various thoughts will flow into your mind when you focus on your breath, and this is normal. Don't think you are doing something wrong just because your mind is not solely focused on your breath.

The one thing you need to get right is circling back to your deep breaths when that focus gets derailed by your interrupting thoughts. If you do that every time, no matter how many times it happens, you are following the procedure of mindfulness meditation. Do it every day for at least fifteen minutes, and you will get better at not being distracted by your thoughts. You will stay focused on your breath alone for a longer period of time; this is where you will become more in tune with what is there.

Chapter 1:

The Ocean

"Can we swim with the dolphins' gain, Mommy?"

"Finish brushing your teeth first!" Jenny called into the bathroom.

The silly child poked her head out of the bathroom, toothbrush in hand, lips covered in toothpaste.

"Okie, Mom!" Flecks of toothpaste flew as she said it and then grinned with foamy teeth.

Kirsty came out, wiping her mouth with the back of her long sleeve, and hopped into the bed as Jenny pulled back the covers.

"I really like the dolphins, Mom. They know how to have fun!"

"They do." Jenny nodded. "But there are all kinds of dreams to explore, you know. There is an entire world full of them out there. All kinds of perspectives you never imagined."

"What does 'perspective' mean, Mommy?"

Jenny tapped a finger to her lips.

"It's... it's a way you view the world. Do you know how you got to see the forest dreaming from the fox's view? That's a new perspective."

"Oh, okay! So what kind of per-spec-tive are we going to see tonight?"

Jenny opened the book, its cover crackling. She flipped through the pages until she came to the next chapter.

"Oh, yes. This is a special one."

She turned the book so that Kirsty could properly see the picture.

It depicted a tropical island, thick with palm trees and ferns, and fallen coconuts on the beach, forming a pattern that looked like the numeral "3."

Above it, in the swaying branches and green canopy, peeked all sorts of brightly colored birds.

Their many calls mingled with the sound of the lapping waves to create a light and hopeful background.

The scent of salt and the pungent fragrance of tropical plants drifted from the pages.

"Now, sweetie, let me show you what the dolphins were so keen to get to explore, but from a different perspective...."

* * *

Jaina woke up on a beach, but not the beach she had left.

Now instead of a sandy path back to the city, she found herself on a tropical island.

Coconuts littered the sand at her feet.

Bright red and spiky fruits hung on some of the trees.

A warm tropical wind blew past, stirring the leaves with a whispering rustle and billowing her hair.

Jaina smiled as she breathed it in. The air smelled so fresh and left a lingering tang on her tongue.

She turned toward the nearby jungle.

A small bird with green feathers and a shiny blue around its head hopped down from one of the branches.

"Welcome!" it chirped. "This is my home. Do you like it?"

Jaina nodded enthusiastically.

"It's wonderful. So warm and cozy and peaceful. How do you ever stay awake here? I think I would spend my day napping if I lived in such a nice place!"

"Oh, but you don't know what else there is to see!" said Bird.

"You would have no time for napping all day if you could see the beauty of this place!"

"Could I? Could you show me?" Jaina looked hopeful, her eyes big and bright.

The bird could not resist her plea.

"Yes, I will show you. Come with me and see what only one on wings can see! Then you tell me if you would spend all day napping."

"Deal!"

Jaina held out her arm, and Bird alighted upon it, tilting its head back and forth to stare at her with each eye.

"And...let the wind takes us!"

Then it flew off again, and Jaina found that she was looking at the beach from high above.

She was like Bird, winging her way through warm blue skies to appreciate the jungle and the ocean from on high.

She circled higher and higher, and the whole island became a green-carpeted seed below her.

They were so high in the sky, only the winds kept them company, singing of the distant waves, of the past and the future.

"Here we go!" Bird dove down, tucking her wings, as the green jungle rushed up to meet her.

She spread her wings and arced smoothly into level flight, circling the treetops.

Below her, she saw the coconuts sitting in the trees, humming softly in the breeze.

Hush voices rose up to meet her: monkeys leaping from branch to branch, picking the fruits and eating them with lyrical delight.

They looked up at Bird as she flew past and waved their hands in envy.

Into the canopy, she plunged.

Green fan-shaped leaves fluttered in the wind as she flew past.

Other birds, some yellow with black beaks, some dark blue with yellow beaks, and still others red with white markings, sang loudly, all competing voices.

They looked up as she flew past. Some rose into the air with a flutter of feathers, but they could not keep up with her speed.

She wove through corridors of green and tan, leaves and branches adorned with fruits or coconuts, nimbly winging around tree trunks, dodging hanging vines, and great big spiderwebs glistening with morning dew like living chandeliers.

The chorus of chirps and hooting cries followed her as she raced through a blur of the jungle.

Then she was free and flew out over the beach, above the water.

Fish leaped and swam in the cerulean waves, all aglow from the sunshine warming the world.

Dolphins cavorted off the shore, leaping high from white-capped waves to glisten in the sun and crash back down again.

Bird Jaina watched the shadows darting about beneath the surface, and then she turned back to the island.

Flocks of seabirds circled on the shores, diving down to peck at some meal washed ashore.

"Food! Food! Food!" their cries said.

The bird had more on her mind than simply eating.

She circled the island, white sand streaming by beneath her, the lush jungle rotating slowly in her eyes.

Slender fingers of sunlight crept through the canopy, and golden dust swirled in their grasp.

Little lizards and dark beetles crawled up the trunks, racing to the top to reach the sunlight. Their voices rose ever higher in competition.

The bird let out a warbling song to drown them out. Her voice echoed in the jungle as she spiraled ever higher, eventually reaching high above the island once more.

"This is an amazing view!" said Jaina.

"Yes, it is." Bird tucked her wings and dove once more.

"But sometimes you need to see from a bird's eye view up close!"

Down she flew into the jungle canopy, landing upon a high branch.

The wind caressed her feathers as she preened her wings and then looked down on the world unfolding below her.

In the thick undergrowth, many creatures crawled, each with a voice of its own.

A furry anteater hummed its slow, ponderous song as it wandered lazily through the brush, long tongue flicking out of its long face.

The anteater stopped and looked up at Bird as she sang down to it.

"Good...morning..." said the anteater, its every word drawn out and rolling.

"It is a good morning!" said Bird. "But there are no ants up here, my friend."

"That's...okay." The anteater plodded along on its search.

A soft croak drew her attention, followed by another and another.

Small frogs with very vibrant coloring hopped up the tree trunk.

Bird knew better than to test them: they were beautiful but dangerous if you were careless, much like the sweetest of dreams.

One of the frogs, neon green with red sides, leaped from the tree as the wind sighed through the palm fronds.

The frog spread into wings of luminous glass, a butterfly with glowing blue and black patterns on its wings.

As Bird and Jaina watched, the butterfly shattered into a hundred tiny slivers of blue light, and each grew wings, a sudden swarm of sky-blue butterflies shining in the shaded forest canopy.

Laughing, Bird flew down to join them and suddenly found herself caught within a cloud of swirling blue.

They spiraled with the wind, down nearly to the ground and then back up into the branches, pushing through the leaves and emerging into the sunlight beyond.

As the butterflies flew, a symphony of fluttering notes filled the air.

The bird stopped flapping her wings and for a moment just drifted up on the music of the island itself: the rush of wings, wind, and waves, all joining together to create a warm sound.

The frond leaves were as wings, emerald feathers joining her in flight.

Whole flocks rose out of the green to take to the sky with her, and they soared so high even the wind envied them.

Blue skies opened up before them, and to Jaina's delight, she found they soared higher still.

Into kingdoms of cloud they flew, where mountains of mist and moisture rolled past, and visions of the ancient world rose up and fell away in mere moments.

Clouds became like islands in the sky, floating upside down in an airy ocean.

The wind rolled through it all like oceanic currents, some warm and lazy, others cool and swift.

The flock changed again, leaves borne upon the wind, now clad in white cloud-feathers, wreathed in a scent of rain.

Thunder rolled, and the islands gave way to a downpour, cascading from the clouds like waterfalls.

The flock dove into the rain, becoming like fish of sea green, fins like wings, but the music never changed— the song of the island: that of sea and sky, where the voices of the waves and the dreams of the wind combined.

Therefore, down they fell, back into the water, bursting through the surface and emerging from a geyser of bubbles in yet another world.

There the deep blue embraced them, warm and salty, and they sank into its liquid softness. Currents enveloped them.

Colorful ocean fish darted back and forth amid the reefs that surrounded the island, and the flock changed yet again, becoming like them, bright and quick, yet trailing seaweed from their tails.

Longer and longer, the trails grew as they flew through the water around the island, binding it in green.

The land became green beneath them, and the clouds of fish were as clouds in the sky glimpsed through the shimmering surface above them.

Green seaweed beds settled onto coral and melted together into trees with palm leaves, and the rocks that once adorned the reef hung from the trees like coconuts.

Sun shone through the surface, upon which the shadows of swaying trees danced.

She landed beside a pool in the center of it all that slowly filled up with clear gleaming water.

The bird looked into the pool, and Jaina was there beside her, staring at their reflections.

She sat back and laughed. "That was amazing!

I never knew the island was so perfectly poised between the two worlds."

"Three," said Bird cheerily.

"Earth, sea, and sky. This little island offers them all for those who want them. Even for one who has hopped and flown every single inch of this island. Do you see now why I never tire of it?

To nap here would be divine, but if this whole place is like a dream come to life, would you need to?"

Jaina sat back on her hands. The warm tropical air stirred her hair and tasted faintly of salt.

She smiled.

"I think it would be hard to tell the difference. This entire place is perfect. As you said, it's got something for everyone."

A coconut fell and rolled down a little sandy hill, bumping lightly into her knee.

Jaina picked it up and found that it already had a straw in it, drawn from the little reeds that surrounded the pool.

She sipped at the sweet coconut milk, the taste rolling over her tongue like the white clouds through which they had flown.

Jaina lay back on a bed of soft, fragrant tropical flowers.

Closing her eyes and just relishing the tastes of the island, Jaina did not even notice the coconut slip from her fingers.

The birds continued their endless cries around her, and the wind continued to caress the waves.

Jaina fell into dreams that had little difference from the waking beauty that was the island life.

Chapter 2:

Fire of Dragons and Flames of Gold

B lood is flowing on the cut on his cheek, flowing down his neck and pooling with tacky perspiration and the violet fix of wounds blooming along his collarbone. His breathing was battered; he fell over, attempting to slow down and rest, to take in what had just occurred. The young man's brilliant brown hair was covered in dried blood, soil, and residue. He looked depleted and harmed; however, she didn't look much better.

Skye inhaled gradually, inclining toward the solid divider and allowing it to hold her as she attempted to lift up her left knee. She panted at the development, gritting her teeth to stop the call of torment. A shapeshifter's claws, a wolf she thought, had caused the long bleeding to expand over her knee in the battle to escape the domain and Academy.

"Skye," The kid sputtered, "Would you say you are OK?"

"Will," She mumbled, "Will, I'm so grieved."

He ventured towards her, his steely dark eyes zeroed in on the pouring cut and the withering young lady before him.

"It's not your shortcoming," Will said immovably, "We were unable to have saved them. Our forces... we scarcely got out in one piece."

Skye covered her face into her hands, attempting to inhale, to quiet down, to stow away as tears pooled toward the edge of her eyes. The essences of Will's family were incredible, agonizing, and playing at the front of her brain. Her kindred understudies at the Academy tumbled to the floor or were meandering around beguiled, attempting to execute each other. All that had occurred just now was unimaginable to her. The adrenalin she had been running on was gone. Skye's capacities as a beginner natural were shot from the psychological and actual weariness of the day. They were undependable over here.

"Skye, would you say you are ready to walk? We need to discover a safe place to stow away to," Will said delicately. The sky was getting dim, and they were with next to nothing, depleted and uncovered, minutes from one of the greatest domain passages into Earth.

Skye lifted her head up, "Definitely, we need to go," She said shakily. The slash in her knee was pulsating. The incident was making her brain fuzzy. "I'll be fine."

Her vision swam before her as she attempted to push through and take care of herself. "Will," She wheezed, "Will, hel-p... " Her eyes rolled into the back of her head as she fell, imploding to the ground in a pile, and faded into oblivion.

The day's events were playing like a highly contrasting tape in her subliminal as Will scooped her up and lifted her behind him, running into the haziness.

The amplifier at the institute was on full blast, ringing in her ears. The frenzy. The study hall abandoning a scene of Celestials calmy concentrating, to the craziness. Her colleagues running and the few that had been entranced, becoming captives of the trespassers and wrapping their hands around Will's throat. The brilliant-haired kid that sat by the window in all of her high-level classes. A talented healer, she had heard. She was unable to run and relinquish him. Her hands turned and sent sparkles of consuming daylight into the knuckles of the strangler's hands. Their hands tumbled from Will's throat; she hollered and proceeded to throw flashes as Will panted for air and fought to his feet.

They had never talked, had never communicated; however, they wouldn't have endured the evening without each other. The passages, he, by one way or another, realized who was beguiled and who was running, thought about where assailants would hop from, and pulled her down to avoid impacts of fire and lines of lightning as they attempted to leave the Academy. What's more, she could pull on her natural force. Daylight started from her hands, blinding the entranced—plants cast from no place, folding over the beguiled bodies and catching them to the floor.

She was in disarray as Will pulled her away from the exit and further into the basement to his family. The turned shifters came after them, wolves and winged serpents obstructing their way. She got to his mom and sister first. Snatching their hands and attempting to ensure them with her body and white-hot daylight safeguard. Will took up the back, an old long blade he'd amassed in a battle grasped firmly, teeth gritted with assurance to get them protected out of here.

The shouting. Spooky, repeating, ricocheting around the stone hallway. The conflicting of swords. The fireballs being grunted from a mythical serpent shifter that got the curve of the entire hall. Flares pursuing them, intensely hot, consuming, rankling, shouting. Running. Fire was all over, and the shifter was all the while coming. Running, running, running until they impacted through the air, tossed against the stone dividers by the blast of blazes turning in a red hot red ball. Missing Skye and Will by meters, however, getting his sister and mom in a mass of red flares. The floor appeared to be flimsy, her ears ringing with shouting, screeching sounds she didn't perceive as her own.

The blood drained from Will's face when he was confronted with the ghastliness and misery as he went into the fire. Skye hurled her arms and sent plants out to get and pull him away. There was nothing they could do.

Staggering out of the institute. Battling, as yet battling to get to the domain access to Earth. To somewhere more secure than here. A shifter snatched and crushed her into the ground. Tearing and tearing. Ear blasting shouts and hollering. Will, smacking the grip of his sword into the shifter's head, pulled her ready for action for the domain section.

Turning, turning, turning, turning, firmly holding to Will. Her fingers braced down on his hands, frozen, frightened, and reeling with insanity. Tumbling out of the passageway and running. Running like she won't ever have. Anguish, her knee giving way as they escaped.

In the murkiness and wellbeing of an abandoned bungalow, Skye's eyelids slid open, pupils enlarged wide with dread and stress.

"Will," She heaved, attempting to move, "Will?"

"Hello, stay there, Skye," He hunkered down next to her, his eyes strangely shocking and moon-like in the black night.

She inhaled, air flowing through her veins, "Where are we, precisely?"

"We're protected," He pressed her hand, "Until further notice in any case. We are in an old cabin, and that's all I know."

"I'm heartbroken," Skye murmured, "Not ideal to pass out when we're running for our lives."

Will gave a dry laugh, "Indeed, it took me a lot to heal you, yet you shouldn't go blacking out on me now."

She grinned. Regardless of the relative multitude of awful things today, she was appreciative to have met him, "Bless your heart. So the bits of hearsay are valid about you being a superb healer for a subsequent year?"

"It appears a portion of the first-years tattle might be correct," He shot back, the trace of a grin lingering on his face.

The light exchange caused them both to feel somewhat better and quiet.

"Do you know why... ?" Skye followed off, lost for words about the circumstance.

Will shook his head, "I have no clue about what just occurred. To start with, we need you to recuperate before we can move to investigate what the heck occurred at the Academy."

Skye gestured and set herself up to take a good look at him. Brilliant twists, penetrating dim eyes, sketchy consumed skin, and wounds, a fragment of where the cut all over had been. No indication of separating, no tears, simply a steely look.

"Are you alright?" Skye investigated his eyes. Dark, consistent, startling,

"I healed myself," He said,

Skye wasn't getting some information about his wounds. Her ardent substantial, and she felt the ghastliness and insanity ascending in her once more.

"Your family," Her lip shuddered as she touched his hand with hers.

He let her hold it, hold him, consoling him in silence.

"I actually have you," Will said delicately, crushing tight.

Chapter 3:

The Danish King

Denmark is high up north, where Germany stops. There is still a king there today, but he is no longer there to govern, but he usually visits kindergartens with his wife because she likes children so much.

But a long time ago, the Danish king was very powerful. As all kings used to do, he always wanted to increase his land so that he would become even more powerful. So he always had to conquer another country. That was not easy. In the south of Denmark was Germany, then the kingdoms of Hanover and Prussia. He could not mess with them because they had many more soldiers than he—likewise, the Swedes, whose country lies close to Denmark.

So he looked north. Far behind the sea was Greenland. This is a huge country, but at the time, it was almost unknown, and it was supposed to be very cold there. So he had three ships loaded from the royal fleet. On each, he put a brave knight and several soldiers, as well as horses and all kinds of war equipment.

They set off to Greenland in the terrible northern cold. When the ships arrived, they first saw a lot of ice and snow. The knights put on their armor and went ashore to conquer it. But they saw no one, and the knights froze in their iron armor on the ice, so they could not move. They kicked wildly, clawing their iron armor hard to free themselves from the ice.

A few of the other soldiers had to make a fire to get them released. As a result, of course, the armor on the feet got pretty hot, and the knights burned their feet. They hopped around wildly until they were finally free and quickly disappeared onto their ships.

Then one tried to bring the horses ashore. He should conquer Greenland. The horses struggled hard, but after a few meters, they also got stuck in the snow. The soldiers could not walk in the high snow, and the cold has merciless. So they finally went with their horses back on the ships. When the knights sat around thinking and pondering, the lookout on the ship's mast reported: "Enemy ahead!!"

And indeed, the knights saw in astonishment how a sleigh was approaching with very small horses. They were even more astonished when they discovered that it was not horses, but many dogs in front of a sled, so effortlessly whizzing across the snow.

Everyone brought their rifles and lances and feared that they would have to defend themselves. But there was only one man on the sled, an Eskimo. He greeted them in a very friendly way and was happy to see so many people because not so many people lived in Greenland, so he often felt quite lonely and alone. He welcomed everyone and asked them if they would not visit him in the evening, his wife would cook a nice soup of seal meat for them.

From whom you are greeted so friendly, you can fight badly against, and so put three of the knights on the dogsled, but without their heavy armor. Husch - you rushed over the landscape to a strange hut, which was made entirely of snow. It's called an igloo and is round, but it's very nice and warm!

When they had eaten, they thanked each other, and the Eskimo drove them back to their ships by dog sled. They then decided to sail back to Denmark.

They then reported everything to the king. He held court with his ministers on how to conquer Greenland. They also asked a wise old man named Count Johannsen. The count whispered his suggestion, to the king's delight, in the ear of the king.

He sent his steward to the city to buy whatever vanilla powder he could get. Then he equipped a ship again, but this time the knights put on thick fur coats and took sleds with them. In addition, the whole load compartment was full of vanilla powder!

Arriving in Greenland, they were greeted by Eskimos again; they were well known by now. Danish soldiers mixed the vanilla powder they brought with clean snow to form delicious vanilla ice cream and gave it to the Eskimos.

They had never eaten anything like that! They were crazy about it and still wanted to have more. The knights, however, kept everything under wraps and first wanted to speak to the Eskimo leader, who was quickly brought for them. With him, the knights made a contract that now Greenland would belong to Denmark, and for that, the Eskimos would get as much vanilla ice cream as they could eat.

Then the knights sailed home with their ship and told their king that Greenland now belonged to Denmark, without there being a war!

And that's how it is today, so you can ask every Dane.

Story Of The Little Annika

I'll tell you the story of little Annika...

Annika pulls her blanket up to her chin, presses her teddy tightly to her, and pinches her eyes. It does not help anything. She escapes night after night to her parents' safe nest. I can understand Annika very well.

What would you say as a parent so that she is not afraid anymore? Would you try to explain to her that there are no ghosts? Annika would protest. They exist very well! She can hear her. Yes, even feel it.

Annika's mother has an idea.

She places a small, green-shining moon in the nursery and tells her daughter, "Do you know that ghosts are afraid of green light?" Annika looks at her mother with wide eyes. "Ghosts are afraid too?" She asks. "Yes, and they cannot harm you when the green moon shines for you."

Annika nods and understands.

Every time Annika hears another giggle or flashes and storms outside, she looks at the moon. She believes in him. Imagines that his green light envelops her, trusts in the wisdom and love of her mother, and closes her eyes calmly.

Ghosts That Adults Fear

However, the story continues...

Annika grows up. At some point, she no longer needs the green light. The idea of witches and monsters is now funny.

However... completely different ghosts appear in Annika's life.

The worry of not finding the right one. The concern that the money for the rent increase is not enough. The fear that she will never fit in her favorite jeans again...

Do you think these ghosts are familiar?

Even thirty years after, she cannot sleep because of ghosts. She turns back to her mother.

"You know, mom, I sometimes lie in bed for hours. The worries just do not want to go away."

"My little one, can you still remember the green moon that drove away all your spirits?"

"Yes. What do you mean by that? A plastic light will hardly be the solution to my worries. These are real!"

Her mother laughs heartily.

"Worries are like ghosts. If you do not believe in them, they cannot hurt you. Because worries or fears have only one power: They keep you from concentrating on what you want.

Your attention is like the headlight of a lighthouse. If it rests on what you want, it cannot be on your worries."

The mother chuckles happily and gets up to leave. She has said everything she needs to say.

You cannot fight worries.

"But mom, if I do not solve my worries, they stay! I have to think about them."

"How did we deal with the ghosts before? Was your closet broken down? Did we trim the feet of your crib or call the Ghostbuster?

No, we did not fight your spirits because they do not exist. Only your attention gave them life. Likewise, your worries only exist in your head. If you try to solve or fight them, they stay alive."

Annika reflects on her mother's words. If a stranger had told her that, she would have labeled him a real refugee. However, she had watched her mother, too many times, keep her smile in any challenge. She never had the feeling that she was hiding something.

"OK," Annika says. "I'll give it a try. But I no longer believe in the protection of the green moon. I'm sorry."

The mother answers. "You have something much, much better. It's your wishes and dreams. Focus your spotlight on the places you see, the people you laugh with, and the successes you want to celebrate.

I promise you that these pictures will come alive every day."

We are faced with choices countless times every day. We can either direct our attention to our concerns or to our dreams.

Our life will be guided by this decision.

Chapter 4:

Coffee House Confession

"Is this seat taken?" asked the young fellow.

"Depends, how do you make a living?" answered the more established lady.

"Uhh- - I'm a film understudy."

"Clever response. You may sit."

"Much obliged, this café is constantly stuffed. I take it you like movies?"

"No doubt, something to that effect. I additionally like understudies."

"I didn't get your name."

"I didn't give it."

"All things considered, my name is Jason. Friends call me Jay."

"I don't shake hands."

"Sorry. I absolutely get it; my mother's a germaphobe, as well."

"You're somewhat charming for a film understudy."

"You know, you're not the first beautiful lady to tell me that. It could be the multi-nutrients I take."

"It could be."

"I took a stab at acting when I was a child, yet they despised that I posed an excessive number of inquiries."

"Like what?"

"Would I be able to go potty? Where's my mom? For what reason doesn't my daddy love me? Stuff like that."

"Is it accurate to say that you are disclosing to me you have daddy issues?"

"It is safe to say that you are interested because we have this trait in common?"

"I'm outraged that you think I have these issues."

"That is to say, don't we as a whole in one way or another?"

"Possibly."

"I never met my father. My mother revealed to me he's an independent movie chief who would prefer to fund-raise for his next film than bring up a kid."

"How does that make you feel?"

"You sound like a psychologist. I trust you're not one. I, as of now, have one of those."

"No, I'm not a therapist. I'm simply a lady in a café."

"An appealing lady in a café. Will your better half show up soon?"

"No."

"Gracious, will your significant other be showing up soon?"

"No. What's more, you didn't respond to my inquiry."

"Um, I don't feel anything. That is to say, you can't actually feel anything for somebody you never knew."

"Would you at any point go search for him?"

"For somebody who will not disclose to me their name, you pose a ton of personal questions."

"Answer my last question and, I'll tell you my name."

"Would I at any point go search for him? Well, probably not. On the off chance that he left, he most likely doesn't have any desire to be found."

"Imagine a scenario where I revealed to you that he's searching for you."

"Your meaning could be a little clearer. Who is?"

"Here's my card. Meet me at this location at 1 p.m. tomorrow. I need to go."

"Pause! You didn't reveal to me your name!"

"Aminah."

"Jason, you're late."

"My class ran late. My bad."

"All things considered, I'm astonished you came by any means. I had the impression yesterday that you would not like to find your dad."

"Truth be told, yet on the off chance that he's searching for me--"

"I sense that you have more interest instead of animosity toward your dad."

"I suppose you can say that."

"Follow me."

"This house is amazing! It reminds me of a scene in Black Mirror. Pause, he's not in there, right? Since I'm here, I can't tell if I need to do this."

"He is, and he's prepared to meet you. In the event that you would prefer not to do this, you're allowed to leave, yet something tells me that you need this."

"How would you find your way into this, Aminah? Is it true that you are his better half? Sweetheart? Realtor? I don't know if I can confide in you."

"Would you be here on the off chance that you didn't confide in me?"

"Truly, you're hot. Like, super-model-hot and oddly enough, I opened up to you at the café about stuff I never thought I'd tell anybody. Presently I'm here, and I feel like for what seems like forever is going to turn over."

"I have that impact on individuals; however, trust me when I say that your life will improve. Kindly follow me."

"Aminah, I need to use the restroom."

"Need to upchuck?"

"Ew, no. For what reason do you believe that?"

"That normally happens when somebody is truly apprehensive."

"I was a child model, remember? My nerves are acceptable. I simply need to go number one truly downright awful."

"The restroom is a few doors down that side. I'll hang tight for you here."

Damn, what have I mixed myself up with? It will not hurt to have a peek around. Gotta ensure I didn't stroll into some mental case's home. I bet she doesn't have the foggiest idea about my father. She said she loves understudies; possibly she brought me here to entice me.

"Aminah found him. No doubt, she brought him here. I don't have the foggiest idea how he will respond. He thinks I deserted him to make motion pictures. OK, that is valid; however, his mom charged me with an assault claim... No, I didn't assault her. It was consensual... I don't have the foggiest idea. She was terrified I planned to leave her for a more youthful entertainer. OK, that is likewise evident, yet I actually reserve the right to know my child!"

"Father?"

"I'll get back to you."

"Who were you conversing with?"

"My dad, uh, your- - your granddad."

"I don't actually have the slightest idea what to do now."

"Can I embrace you?"

"Of course, I presume."

"Amazing, you're a major person now, huh?"

"Much obliged?"

"Take a load off. Do you need anything to drink? Water? Espresso? Wine? Whisky? I could use a glass myself."

"No, I'm good. How do you know Aminah?"

"She's an old companion. She has some expertise in discovering individuals. She disclosed to me you're a film understudy?"

"Yes."

"Am I the reason?"

"Possibly."

"I don't know what your mom told you- - "

"Her form of reality."

"Right."

"I didn't come here for a present or anything. I only wanted to know what you looked like."

"Also,

"No big surprise, mother takes a gander at me in an unusual manner when she's had lots of wine."

"Gracious, your mom is an incredible lady. I was beguiled by her, yet we wanted different things."

"I'm sorry she had me."

"No! Never say that! Your mother needed - we needed you so terrible."

"Why didn't you stay?"

"At that point, coordinating motion pictures appeared to be simpler for me than parenthood."

"Was it awesome?"

"This will sound truly wrecked to you; however, yes, it was great."

"No, I get it. Follow your dreams or raise a family, yet you can't have both."

"Precisely, you comprehend."

"I likewise see every one of the evenings mother cried on the grounds that she was distant from everyone else without hearing a word from you and every one of the occasions she was tanked calling me by your name and cussing me out."

"I'm sor- - "

"Try not to apologize. I disclosed to Aminah yesterday that I don't feel anything with regards to you since I never knew you. Subsequent to meeting you today, I'm more than OK with that."

"Child, if you at any point need anything- - "

"I have myself and my mother. I'll see myself to out."

"Jason! Come back, Jason!"

"Much appreciated, Aminah, for the entirety of this. You're correct; my life is improving."

"Will you see your dad once more?"

"No, however, I desire to see you again at the café for more conversation."

Chapter 5:
The Eagle Takes You with Him

Before we begin this journey downwards into the deepest realms of our subconscious, let us take a minute to physically and mentally and spiritually acclimate ourselves into being aware of our inner sanctum and internal workings. We will begin by going to a place of comfort, ideally a bed or a very comfortable reclining chair, and we will relax our bodies to the furthest extent possible. Now, close your eyes, staying firmly on your back, with your arms relaxed at your sides and your legs rested downwards. Take one deep breath in, through your nostrils, counting slowly to four, and one deep breath out, through your nostrils again, counting slowly to four. Breathe in the breath of the spirit and breathe out the stress of the day. Now is the time to rest. Become aware of nothing but the air flowing through your nostrils, envision a steady flowing stream, smooth inhalations, and exhalations, let your body become weightier and more relaxed with each passing cycle of breath. Allow your thoughts to become completely still, as you focus on your core, your solar plexus, allowing your thoughts to flow outwards past your vision until they escape your being, while only holding and retaining the pure awareness of spirit, the holy serenity of the mind and body. Breathe in, one, two, three, four, then breathe out, one, two, three, four, each breath becoming slower. One... two... three... four... One... two... three... four... One... two... three... four... One... two... three... four... One... two... three... four... One... two... three... four... Continue this pattern of breath, expanding, and sink down deeper into yourself, becoming a voyeur of your own still, relaxed body, lost in time. Become lost in this experience as you journey further into the trance, and prepare for the road we are about to embark upon. Draw further and further away from your still, lying body and into the realm of imagination, where images grow, the land of dreams that you are about to become one with. Erase your mind of all that is within it currently, and prepare the landscape for a new and fresh experience in the farther reaches of reality. One... two... three... four... inhale... One... two... three... four... exhale... One... two... three... four... inhale... One... two... three... four... exhale... Now, with your mind, body, and spirit rested totally, entranced, and fertile, let us begin.

It seems as if all of the earth is on fire, dry, deserted land stretched out as far as the eye can see, gone up in flames. You don't look down, but you can almost feel the heat on your legs, or maybe that's just your imagination. You are clutched to your guardian, soaring through the sky, his generous, unlimited bounty of feathers molding to your frame, providing a cushion, providing a grip, providing a shelter. He soars down, and you lose your stomach, he soars up, and you feel a slight pullback, but know that he would never let you fall; this giant, glorious

44

eagle that saved you from that mountain peak just before the flames engulfed it, now carrying you to some isolated safety that only he knows. You feel you are working in total tandem with this creature, you called him forth from deep inside, and he came from the outside to take you upon him. He flew down and beckoned to you, and you perched atop him and set forth into the night, leaving behind the dangers of the world. Now you are soaring, possibly across the furthest reaches of the globe. It has been an incredibly long journey, but you are in the best company. You would be totally satisfied to never let go. Being here is like being at home, in bed, dreaming, in the most finely fluffed pillows and comforters with the smoothest silk sheets. For all you know, this could be a dream and one that you never wake up from. The two of you converse, in silent thoughts and feelings flowing from your skin into his feathers at the point of contact, and back to you when he is done with them, improving on them, giving you all that he has to offer, in his grand and glorious wealth of spirit. Is this creature even real? Is this some God? For all intents and purposes, it might as well be. This is heaven, this is your guardian angel, and you are flying the greatest heights ever known to man. You hug the beast and caress your face against his feathers. A great love is brought forth in this vibration, from your cheek to his feathers and into his being and vibrating outwards back to you. He tells you everything is going to be okay. "You are safe here, and now, you will always be safe with me, and I will always be there to protect you," he says. You ask the eagle where he is taking you, and he answers that he is taking you where you want to go. You don't know where that is. But in the greater language that the two of you are sharing, maybe this message is as plain as day. You feel as though you are open books to each other and awakening in each other new things just by sharing in the exposure. This creature sees you, and feels you, and knows you, like a family member, like a spirit watching you, like a guardian angel. The journey is long, eternal. You have been flying seemingly across the galaxy and have lost track of time due to the incredible comfort and peace, and serenity gained from your new companion, which has totally relaxed your mind and its perceptions. This may as well be the destination unto itself, and this journey might as well continue on for the rest of your lifetime. The grip of your body onto his back is like the completion of a puzzle, as if you have met your maker and are now having a personal conversation with God himself. You wonder where the beast came from, if he was manifested at the exact moment you needed him, if he had always been there, connected to you, or if he is just another life, alongside yours, that happened to coincide with your own at this time, just so happening to provide you with the strongest bond that you have ever felt. You ask him. His answer seems to just say that he is here now, and that is all that matters. Maybe he does not know. Maybe it just doesn't matter. This eagle is a bridge between you and eternity, for in him you feel your eternal self, as well as a connection to something greater. Even if he were to fly back to earth and put you down wherever that may be, you would still be with him, flying here, for a long, long time. Maybe forever. This is something that will never leave you, this experience, now that it has been granted. You have been given the gift of flight, now, through this being. Wherever you are, you will always be in heaven. You brace yourself and raise your head to peer over the great beast's shoulders. You can see the curve of the earth forming at the horizon. Whatever it was of the smoke seems to have dissipated, the flames now long, far off behind you. Maybe the world wasn't on fire after all; maybe it was just that mountain. You can't be so sure of anything right now. Somewhere, out there, is home. You don't remember. But he knows. He knows where you belong, and he is taking you back. You realize that at this moment, whatever happened, you don't know yourself. You could be anything or anyone, and your greatest identification at this moment is with the beast. The horizon is giving away to what looks to be an ocean, a body of water that is stretching out further than you can define. The eagle is heading straight into it. The wilderness of the land is giving way to the shore; what once was a sprawling sea of trees breaks up intermittently to become a sprawling sea of blue oblivion. The entire atmosphere changes, and the heat turn into a pleasant, breezy coolness. Is this where your home is? Is your home past this ocean? Maybe among the ocean, on a small, secluded island? Is it a home you know or a home you

47

are about to meet? As you breach the shore, the eagle swoops down, and you become very close to the water. He wants to cool you off. He wants you to see the glimmering light of the stars reflected off this gorgeous mirror. A billion little twinkles, a labyrinth of lights, stretched out as far as the eye can see. Then he soars back up, and, with that, you are hypnotized. You close your eyes, and you are flying through the stars themselves, alone; you are channeling this beast, and he is within you, but you are alone. You are flying and flying, and it will never stop. You feel so relaxed, your body falls out of itself, there is only light, forever, a million light-years through space, a never-ending journey through the rivers of time, and you are asleep.

Chapter 6:

Lost City in the Woods

"As I read this and begin to drift comfortably asleep, I don't know whether I will find myself drifting asleep more to the sound of my voice or the words I read or perhaps to the spaces between the words. And as I drift comfortably asleep, I'll just read this story to myself."

So, as you listen to me, you can begin to drift comfortably asleep, and while you begin to drift comfortably asleep, you can allow yourself to get comfortable and allow your eyes to close. And I don't know whether you will drift off to sleep with the words that I use, with the sound of my voice, or perhaps with the spaces between my words.

And you can have a sense of being out bird-watching one day, of being in a little shed, a little bird-watching shack, with some binoculars gazing out from this quiet spot. You are gazing out through some woodland, over a large valley, and you can see different birds in the nearby bits of woodland, but you can also see a large circling bird of prey in the distance in the valley, and you can see it so gracefully circling. Seeming to use almost no effort and you look through binoculars at that graceful bird of prey, and you have that unusual experience where, when you watch that through binoculars, you shut off from the reality around you and awareness of the shack and awareness of everything else, to almost like you are very near to the bird, almost flying with them.

And while you continue to fly gracefully, you start exploring. And it is as if somehow you have taken over this bird. And a part of you is thinking, "Am I still in the shack watching the bird and have somehow have drifted into a daydream, or was I watching the bird so intensely that I have got into the bird's psyche, somehow managed to get into the bird's mind?" And either way, you go with the experience.

You feel a sense of elegance and grace, and you continue exploring. And you are now in an area you have never been before. As a bird watcher, you have been and watched birds before. You have even been down and walked through the valley, you have even walked and seen some of that river and the lake, but now you seem to have flown over an area you have never been before. An area of woodland, only you notice something about this woodland.

Your eyesight is so good that you notice subtleties; you notice that some trees are slightly higher up than others, and notice there is a certain pattern to these trees, and intuitively something tells you it is worth going down there and investigating.

So you fly down, but you are too big to fit through the treetops in this area of the woodland, so you circle around and explore and conclude that you are going to have to land at the beginning of the woodland, but you don't know how well a bird of prey is going to be able to walk from the beginning of the woodland all the way into the woods. You don't see an alternative, so you fly around and land at the entrance of the woodland, and as you come in to land, you bring your wings back, you open them wide, slowing you right down, catching as much wind as possible, catching as much of that air as possible.

And you put your feet out in front of you, and you have an odd experience, that just as your feet touch the ground, you become yourself again, and you find yourself standing before the woodland. You are still trying to work out whether this is a dream and whether you have somehow gazed at that bird so intensely that you are now dreaming and having this experience, and yet it feels very real and undream-like. And you think, if it was just a dream, wouldn't you just wake up by just deciding this is a dream and just wake up and yet it doesn't seem like a dream or something you can wake up from. It's not something that bothers you; it is just curiosity.

You walk into the woods, listening to the footsteps, listening to the different sounds in the woods, noticing how the light changes as you walk into the woods. The woods are quite dense, and you have to push and work your way through. And as you push and work your way through the woods, you notice that there are some areas that seem to be a bit higher and others that seem to be a bit lower, like the woods have built on top of something. But you don't know what, and you keep pushing and pushing until eventually there is an area that is a little bit clearer, and you notice that the woods have overgrown over some kind of old building. And as you walk around and explore, you find that it seems to have grown over lots of old buildings.

You keep walking and keep exploring, and all you keep finding is more and more buildings like this is a huge area of many buildings. Then you find a bit that looks like a normal bit of land, perhaps a normal outcrop of rock, and you decide to go and explore it, and you scratch through the plants that have covered it over, and you notice that it is a wall of a building that has partially collapsed.

You follow this wall to see where it leads. It seems like you have found some kind of building that would have been near the center of this lost city. Then as you keep exploring, you notice an indentation in the ground, and you notice that this is where an entrance must have once been. So, you start clearing this entrance space, and you find that just behind a bit of rubble is a tunnel heading downwards with some steps.

You walk into the tunnel, and as you do, somehow, oddly, your eyes adapt to be able to see in this tunnel, like somehow you have got some of the abilities of the wild animals in this area. You don't try to understand it because you are too busy thinking that it benefits what you want to achieve— you want to explore this area. So, you head down deeper into this building. And quite a way down, you find a stone slab that you think is probably blocking an entrance to something. And you start pushing around on the stone slab and around on the wall around the stone slab, and then somehow, you just take a step, and the slab moves aside. It grinds and moves aside as you walk through, and you find yourself in a vast chamber.

You read the scroll with fascination, with wonder, only vaguely aware of the positive impact it is going to have on you. And you read that this one also includes instructions saying that all the scrolls can be read when held on this pedestal by this golden clasp. So, you go and get another scroll, you place that on the pedestal and clasp it into place, and you watch as the writing transforms, almost like mist and movement and changing of the text, to become readable. And you read that one, and it is full of knowledge you never would have known, ancient knowledge, ancient wisdom. Then you get another scroll, putting that one back, and notice that that scroll also contains ancient wisdom. And you wonder how long it would take to work your way through the thousands of scrolls full of ancient wisdom in this place.

You read scroll after scroll. Taking in and learning more ancient wisdom. Learning on an instinctive level. Learning that with a certain focus, you can become the animals, you can join the spirit of the animals, and somehow you had stumbled across that focus and by stumbling across that focus, allowed you to stumble across this knowledge. And you read and learn and find this knowledge fascinating. And you realize it would take too long to learn all of this knowledge right now, you decide to continue exploring. And so, you put the original scroll back in place on the pedestal and make sure all the other scrolls are put away in their places, and you explore deeper and deeper into this space.

And as you explore, so you discover a giant underground lake and on that lake is a boat, and this lake is totally still, and you feel it is so still that it is almost unnaturally still, but then, there is no breeze down here. Then you see a puzzle on the wall, and you know there is no further to go in this chamber, but you think it is curious having a puzzle, so you try and solve the puzzle. And after a while moving things around, trying to work the puzzle out, suddenly you get the puzzle, something inside you clicks and makes it make sense to you, and then a secret door opens.

You go through the secret door, going deeper and deeper into this building. And you see a room so large that you can't see the other side of it. You can't see the side on the left or the side on the right. You don't know how the ceiling is being held up in a room this large. And you walk into the room, and after a very, very long time of walking in a straight line so that you don't get lost, just following the markings on the ground, you find yourself at another pedestal, only on this pedestal is a bit confusing, you see a perfectly polished black pebble.

You continue to find your way out and then find your way into the woods. Then you work your way through the wood, back the way you came, and when you exit the woods, you don't know how far it is to get back to where you came from. You know you are supposed to be bird-watching, but you don't know how to get back to where you are bird-watching. And then you feel this compulsion to jump. And you jump up in the air and instantly, you seem to have wings, and you do a large flap and launch yourself higher into the air, and you notice you are that bird again and you fly and catch an updraft of warm air and you spiral round and rise up higher into the air.

You don't give it any thought; you just seem to know your way back to where you were first seen as a bird, and you fly your way back to that location and circle around in that location, and the next minute you feel a slight curious feeling and realize you are looking through some binoculars at the bird and you wonder whether that was all a dream and are curious what it was all about. Then you look down and notice you have a pebble in your shoe and realize it wasn't all a dream. Something happened, some experience, and you don't know what it all means, and you decide to follow those instructions of keeping that pebble in your shoe until such a time as it is just naturally time to lose the pebble. And so that is what you decide to do.

Chapter 7:

The Rejected Woman

He was the perfect man, she met him at one of his jobs. When they met the first time, the crush was immediate, they began to talk, and you could feel the connection, the desire to know each other, and the taste they had. It wasn't difficult to meet for the first date and also for the first kiss to come up, which happened in the middle of that first date.

The desires of the flesh were also present, he let them appear, and she also let go of some garments, but she did not allow it to happen, sex on the first date, no. Abby was a decent girl and would not allow it, no matter how much she wanted to. She was able to hold out until the third, where she accepted his fifth invitation to her house, taking advantage of her parents' absence.

The first meeting was one of those magical ones that take place between couples who seem to know each other from a past life, no matter how many people they have been with, that is the ideal one, and no one surpasses it.

The connection from then on became deeper. They started dating formally; she took him to meet her parents at a Sunday dinner, he brought her back home when the parents had already returned from a trip, and both families were fond of each other.

He would help with the Sunday barbecue at Abby's house and talk about cars with his father-in-law, and she would talk with her mother-in-law about the church, dating issues, and even her jobs when they were visiting.

It was no surprise when the courtship was made more solid with an engagement ring he gave her that belonged to her grandmother, then her mother, and now her.

She started a job in a textile company, where she took the administrative position, her career, and he had now changed to a business where he would have to do multilevel, although the company of this service was extremely strange, he had never heard of the company. But this one promised juicy profits for him, so he entered.

From the moment he entered that company, the boyfriend changed completely, he stopped being the same loving man he had always been, although he treated Abby well, it seemed that every one of his acts was fake, he felt forced to make every gesture, every word of love and even during sex, where they used to be very compatible., now it was a relationship where she felt used, and when it was over she didn't feel full, full of pleasure and protected by the warmth of her man's love, no, now she felt empty, with a strange depression, like when you have sex with a stranger at the disco and the next day you have a moral hangover.

She begged him a thousand times to explain what was going on, but he said everything was fine, he filled her with words of love, he spoiled her and Abby believed him, she had to do it, and they returned to the tense calm where every day they were distancing themselves.

The date of the marriage was getting closer, her mother had made the preparations, they had looked for a wedding dress, the trousseau, the borrowed, stolen, blue, and everything was ready to have it that day. Her fiancé was very excited; he also said he was preparing everything.

When the marriage was one week away, he called her and asked her to come on Wednesday, three days before the wedding, to St. Simons, Georgia, because he had to tell her something. This is one of the Golden Islands. She is full of doubts and waits anxiously and with the hope that she could recover her fiancé and return to what they were.

Those days were painfully long, because in passing her boyfriend almost didn't call her, when the day finally came she appeared in this romantic town, just where she always saw herself with her boyfriend when they went a few times in the past, and there he stood.

They hugged for a long time, more because of her, who was so happy to have him by her side, to feel him, to smell him. Finally, when they broke apart, he looked at her with a smile, that smile that she loved so much, and told her that they should talk.

—We must talk about something important.

—What do you want, my love?

—We are not getting married.

Abby's face was one of bewilderment and the beginning of a breakup that fragmented her into very small pieces.

—I don't understand what you're talking about.

—The company needs me in India, where it is based. I'm leaving tonight, so I won't be able to marry you.

What could have been expected happened, she cried and complained, and he told her that it was the best thing for her career, if when he returned they still loved each other, then they could get married, but the man's attitude already showed the lie, he had simply changed it for his career and that love he claimed to profess had been a farce.

Abby returned with her soul torn apart. At home, she cried for many hours, hugging her pillow, biting it, shouting insults, screaming his name.

She had suffered for love, but never for one where she was at the door of the altar, so close to the one she believed to be the love of her life, and now she would have to throw everything away, she did not understand the attitude of her fiancé. What had happened to him? How could he leave without marrying her? Why did he not invite her to India? She would have followed him to the end of the world because she loved him.

Her parents tried to encourage her, but they were not successful, every day was the same as the day before, without bathing, she went to the bathroom, saw herself in the mirror, ugly, untidy, and crying, eating reluctantly what they put in her mouth, just enough not to die of starvation. Her friends came to see her, but she won't receive them. She just stayed in bed all day, reminiscing about what happened, feeling and wondering what she had done wrong, blaming herself, replaying scenes, words she said, messages, trying to find out what she did to make the love of her life choose a company over her.

Some days she began to check his networks, read the messages that were exchanged on Facebook, those of WhatsApp, interpreting his words, also his own.

Little by little, she began to feel that deep sadness, moving to mild anger, sometimes towards herself, but others towards her ex-boyfriend. She read all the conversations again and remembered the scenes they took place in, remembered her body language, and felt that there were things that did not fit, that words were slipping through the cracks, and were not as honest as she could have expected.

Then she began to see, to realize that she had been stupid, blind, like all women in love and that she was the only one who wanted to get married, that soon after they got engaged the changes began to take place and she had not opened her eyes to the fact that her man's attitude had changed and she had not realized it, that she seemed to use her cell phone more, details that her brain found an explanation for, but that now made sense. The man had backed down after asking for the engagement. Her man had changed his mind; he didn't want anything formal with her and didn't want to be imprisoned in the marriage. But she was so in love and hadn't realized it.

The day she discovered that she was not guilty, that her love had been honest, she felt great relief. It was a strange sensation, like when you get a bullet in the head and you do not feel pain, but you feel a daze. That day she took a long bath and came out renewed, went to bed, and slept well, without nightmares. The next day she went down to eat, and her parents did not say anything, but she saw the joy on their faces; their daughter had come out of the abyss.

For several weeks she was around the house, did not talk much, spent her afternoons by the window, drinking chocolate, and reading, immersed in her thoughts, reflecting, and every day a little more responsive.

A month later she decided to go out, a friend invited her for a coffee, and she said yes, she dressed in jeans, a simple blouse and went to see her, they talked all afternoon, her friend tried to get information from her about the breakup, but Abby was emphatic that she did not want to talk about it, so they started talking about everything, except love.

Little by little, Abby returned to her life again, she found another job. She was fired from the former one because she had abandoned it. She spent several months going to work and returning home, always feeling in her mother's nest all the security she needed.

But one day, finally, after so much pain, so much sorrow, Abby felt free of sadness. She could already think about her love relationship and felt neither anger, nor pain, nor sadness. She wanted neither good nor bad for her ex; he was like a simple stranger. The broken relationship was an experience not to be repeated. She was ready to return to her life, to return to her dreams and now renewed, a new version, where she learned lessons and knew how to love herself first before others over her.

One day, in a meeting of friends at the house of one of her best friends, a man approached her, nice, with the evident intention of flirting, she was opened up the options, she was ready to want something again, but always keeping her guard up, she would pass through that horrible experience. Never again.

Chapter 8:

A Rainy Day

T he downpour was heavy, I had no umbrella, yet ye, I love getting wet in downpours. The sky was dark with mists, and the petrichor brought wistfulness.

"Venti!!!" I knew the voice.

It was Tash, with an umbrella.

"Hello, Tash!"

"Venti, ye come here, don't get cold once more."

"Ye much obliged, I see you got an exceptionally huge umbrella."

"Yea, to help companions from getting cold."

"Ye, much obliged; likewise ye, don't call me Venti, my present moniker is Siva."

"You do have a great deal of nom de plume, haha," another recognizable voice.

"Sophie! Goodness! Howdy!" I got eager to see another dear companion.

"Goodness, howdy Sophie! What an astonishment!" Tash grinned.

"Ye, I brought your umbrella, Tash, and great to see you both!"

As we were talking, The water from rooftop tops ran open into the road. Small children with waterproof coats emerging from the school with guardians, strolling through the puddles out and about. The sound of water drops and the example of waves they shaped when they hit the puddles were fascinating.

So three of us were strolling under a single umbrella, having a decent talk, and Sophie needed to get hot espresso. Hot espresso of Downspring is one of the amazing things that makes this spot what it is.

"It was particularly wonderful to see both of you," I said as I began to taste the hot espresso.

"Yea same, I came here for an evening walk, and it abruptly started to rain," Sophie said

"Yea, glad to see you as well, and yea, the climate is eccentric," Tash said.

Downspring, a particularly delightful spot; I have a ton of companions here, Tash, Sophie, Serena, Lavender, Jooshy, just to mention a few.

Also, the city consistently was a decent home to me; it still is.

I love it so much, drinking hot espresso in a downpour with companions, chilling by the lake, and passing through the spotless roads around evening time; what else can one ask for?

As we talked, the downpour started to cool off and stopped altogether, giving room for the sun to rise.

"Aight," I said, "It was great conversing with you both, Tash and Sophie; however, I need to go now, duty calls, see ya!"

"See ya, Siva! Fare thee well! Bye"

Thus I left the bistro and advanced toward Townsquare.

Townsquare, it's a dim structure with a dull past with me.

I generally despised the spot. It's one reason why I need to leave the city; however, I do have many things I love here and a ton of companions. Was that a great explanation? I truly don't have the foggiest idea; that is the reason I am constantly befuddled about whether or not to the city.

As I approached, my recollections run a streak.

###

"Heya Jooshy!!!"

"Hello, Venti!!! Down for a game?"

"Sure!!"

"Lemme attempt the four-stage registration, hehe," I thought Jooshy was too brilliant and handily hindered it, haha. We were genuinely playing it while the children were going near.

Ten minutes passed, and Jooshy had the high ground; I was thinking and thinking, and unexpectedly, one of the children ran upon our chessboard. BOOM!!!

The child was short and keen-looking. He gazed at us with dread until we both burst out laughing, and he chuckled with us as well. "Be cautious next time!" we grinned and advised him to play with care; he grinned back and went to play.

"In this way, it's a draw, hehe'" I said.

"Fine, haha."

As we were talking, we heard a tremendous commotion. Townsquare was falling.

"Good gracious," Jooshy said, "Go get the children!"

We both ran and took the children in our arms and raced to the steps. The structure was tumbling down onto us.

A gigantic piece of the roof fell and hindered our way down.

"Be Fast! Go through the little opening, children!" I said.

We have figured out how to get two of them on the opposite side safe; however, a greater amount of the roof started to fall and shut the opening.

The brilliant-looking child, Jooshy, and I were trapped.

"The structure's going to fall totally whenever."

"What will we do now?"

"Hear me out, Jooshy. There is an emergency exit on the opposite side."

"In any case, that way is blocked as well."

"I can hold it long enough till-"

"No! I will hold it; your arms should be stinging."

"Ahh, however "

"Trust me, I will fare better."

"I believe in you-"

Thus, he lifted the bar obstructing our path, it opened the way, and we could see individuals surging down the crisis exit.

"Quick!" Jooshy said, and I rushed with the kid. It was so dusty surrounding us, and I at long last came out and could see unmistakably, there were many individuals going down through the emergency exit. I gave the child to a woman there and hurried to go for Jooshy, yet as I turned the side, the floor started to fall, and the man remaining close to me got my hand, "There's no going there,"

"Be that as it may, old buddy, he's stuck there..."

"I'm heartbroken; however, there's no way around it currently. We should simply trust he gets by," as he said, he walked me into the ground floor...

###

Townsquare- three years after that episode- It's been reconstructed into something different, yet it won't ever lose the smell of the lives it took away.

As I proceeded with my stroll to my office, I saw the dividers which we painted together, presently dormant... The streets we strolled together, presently I am strolling alone... what the city took from me, I will detest it until the end of time... the spots we went together... presently it feels forlorn...

As I strolled, I attempted to not see anything, the spots around, and after a long walk, I arrived at my office, another dim structure...

"Congratulations, Siva!!" Everyone began to cheer.

"Umm?Thanks?"

"You got a promotion!"

"Heavenly stars," I thought, a promotion? Ye, that is exceptionally sudden.

"Your new office is in Gladz."

"Wha-?"

"You generally needed to leave this city, ye now's the time!"

Gracious yea, I needed to leave it so terribly, the city, all that it took from me, old buddy, my family, my... With each one of those recollections all over the place, it's simply so difficult to remain here.

I left to the advanced specialty of tall structures, towers, expedient vehicles, and the dim environment...

I remained there. I was certain that would be the last time I would be seeing this, so I took a good look at them with open eyes after quite a while; what a lovely city, and yet, what a revolting city.

"Sir!" I heard a natural voice.

I thought back and knew who it was.

It was Serena in her vehicle.

"Serena!" I shouted in fervor.

"How are you, dear sir?"

"Long time no see! Also, I am fine!"

"Ye, you do appear to be energized, sir."

"Indeed, madame," I showed her my promotion letter.

"Goodness, congratulations! I'm so glad for you!"

"Much obliged to you! By the way, when did you come here?"

"Goodness yea, the work for which I went to Mauriseas is done; thus I am back ye."

"Gracious, and I will leave soon ahh... I truly wish I spent more time with you."

"It's fine. You're not simply leaving this spot perpetually. You will return, right?"

"I don't think so..."

"Why?! You have a ton of companions here, Venti."

"However, a ton of haters too, you know, and many things that frequently annoy me..."

"In any case, contrasted with individuals that adore you, they are so few."

"Be that as it may - ye, never mind about it, how was your time in Mauriseas?"

We talked for like ten minutes, and Serena got a call, so I bid her farewell, and I started thinking, "what am I abandoning here?"

Not simply awful recollections and scorn... but also the affection and the sweet memories.

I started strolling once more, to the spots with each one of those recollections, my companions ye, I do have misconceptions with them, yet eventually, we as a whole social affair, presently I need to leave them.

I strolled through the ringer road, recollecting each memory I had there with my companions, I treasured them, yet now I need to go, correct?

As I strolled, I met Lavender. The day was loaded up with shocks I was unable to think, meeting all companions, and furthermore an advancement, I started to contemplate whether it was a fantasy.

"Lav!" I waved!!

"Spects!" she waved and came strolling quickly towards me.

"How are you?"

"Of course, what about you, borthah?"

"Goodness yea, I am fine, ye just befuddled sista."

"Gracious, about what?"

Thus I told her as well, and she was glad I got a promotion, and yet, she became miserable when I said I ain't returning.

What's more, if ever you are pondering, ye Spects, Siva, Venti they are for the most part my names, I use a lot of names haha, that is the reason.

I realized it was getting late and considered returning home when abruptly it started to rain.

Indeed, it poured heavily once more, and you know what? I had an umbrella this time, yee!! I opened it and started strolling, and as I was going, I saw somebody.

"Hello, Tash!" I called

She was getting wet in the heavy downpour as she was strolling. She looked back and said, "Hello, Siva."

I immediately went to her to cover her with my umbrella, "Don't get wet," I said.

And afterward, we started to talk about the promotion stuff, and she said, "Do what you want to do, Venti, I will be disturbed."

Well, yea, she didn't advise me to stay, nor go, that was a backhanded method of advising me to not leave, her direction, and as we strolled, I started recollecting the days of yore.

"Tash, you recall? Your disunity username is "downpour," you love downpour. I always wanted to ask why but forgot, now I am asking, for what reason do you adore downpour?"

"Ok, well, "downpour" is a cool word, and I wish it was my genuine name; and furthermore, tuning in to music while it downpours is very satisfying. Thank you for coming to my ted talk. The end."

I giggled when she said ted talk and quickly covered it up with a cough, "That is so cool; I do cherish downpour as well. It's simply so lovely like you."

Damn, haha, I didn't have a clue what to say, so I said that, and now she's blushing. We soon get to her house.

"Farewell, Siva!"

Thus I began strolling alone once more; however, the downpour stays with me like a partner, the sound, the chillness, the sensation of water sprinkling over your feet; it was simply so stunning.

Tash and I were old buddies, yet then we had made a lot of mistakes as well, and for the majority of it was my fault, yet false impressions are normal in companionship, correct?

Each one of those senseless things and battles, I figured, I would miss them all so much, and yet, the city will consistently remind me whenever I go through those spots... I was in a predicament, and I strolled through the recreation center; out of nowhere, I heard a sound.

I ran towards it. I recognized who it was but was still pleasantly surprised. I shouted as I saw the face, "JOOSHY!!!!!!"

Chapter 9:

The Ocean Sings

Y ou are on a small remote island. The sand and ocean are pristine, the vegetation is full and lively. Simple living may be a way of life here, and it looks like time itself passes slower. There's no hurrying about as you opt to go for a walk on the fantastic beach. The sun is low in the sky; the air is warm and excellent. The glistening sand is soft, almost white in color, as your feet sink slowly and softly into the nice and cozy, welcoming sand with each step. Allowing the heat to spread around your feet but not stick as you gracefully stroll along the water's edge. The water to your right may be a beautiful Caribbean blue, with white foam bubbles because the waves gently caress the beach.

As you slowly walk, you hear the ocean; seeming to swell in the great distance, but when it reaches you, it's a whisper. A remnant of the good wave it once was. If the ocean were an individual, what things could it tell you? Wouldn't it tell you of its survival and of its suffering? Of the astounding life it provides for many? Wouldn't it sing it in a song? Hear the ocean. Are you able to hear it sing? Is it a sweet lullaby? Is it singing ever softly? As you watch the waves dancing to the song, you yearn to feel them caress your skin. Walking just barely into the water, you feel the wave crash upon your tired feet.

Feel the sand beneath you subside because the earth pulls you down. Stand still; allow the ocean to embrace you. The coolness of the water quickly passes because the wave surrounds your ankles, allowing your feet to sink just a bit further into the nice and cozy sand. While the water sways out, you feel your body call it back to return. It does, it always does. The water goes out; it comes back in. The ocean breathes, just like you. The water comes in; you take a deep breath, filling your lungs with oxygen. You exhale, the water rushes out, carrying that sweet oxygen from your head right down to your emerged toes. Hear the ocean's song because it breathes with you, swaying with the gentle sounds, settling your body down into the world. Just like the roots of a tree, you're beneath the world now while still reaching for the sky, anchored into the life-giving solid base of this planet.

You hear a giggle in the distance, instantly recognizing the tinkling sound of a young child playing on the beach. Such pure joy and happiness call to you. As you approach the kid, you receive a warm welcome. They giggle and continue in their little world of happiness. Slightly ahead, there's a bench. You opt to take a seat for a short time and just enjoy the scenery, the sun low over the ocean, the palm trees behind you swaying with the sunshine breeze. The sand is soft and warm and glistening the reflection of the sun. You lay your head back, allowing your neck to relax as you listen to the sounds. The ocean is singing its song because it breathes in and out. The child is giggling with pure joy and happiness. This place is paradise; it's as if there's no room for the cloudy thoughts of tomorrow and the doubts in the recesses of your mind; all of your troubles escape.

You feel a soft tap on your shoulder and open your eyes to see the sweet child smiling at you. The kid hands you a container of bubbles. Without speaking any words, you recognize this child is asking you to blow the bubbles for him. You feel silly, twiddling with this child, but there's no harm. You open the bubbles, dip the wand, and exhale gently. A stream of iridescent bubbles spews forth. The kid giggles and dances as they fall around them. You feel yourself smile; knowing the very simple effort you put forth caused somebody else such great joy is a rewarding sensation. You repeat a couple of times, but the child's parent is looking for him. He abruptly runs away; you are trying to call him back to give the bubbles back, but he's gone.

Left alone with your thoughts and the child's play, you speak to your inner child. "What does one want in life?" You ask it. As your mind responds, you blow an enormous, soft bubble and watch it touch the ground. Your mind is settled making the exchange; a bubble is simply nearly as good as a solution on this island. Anything that's on your mind, make it into a bubble and blow it away. Regardless of how big or small, each bubble is satisfied to be left alone. Collect each thought you have, pour them into this bubbling liquid. Dip in the wand, and blow all of them away. This is often some form of relaxation. Nothing stands in your way except your mind. Who controls your mind? Control each thought as you make consistent, beautiful bubbles. Watch them drift over the ocean, carrying your troubles far away from you.

Watching the bubbles disappear over the ocean, you notice the sun is now even lower in the sky. There's still no rush, nothing to hurry to, nothing to stress you; simply be and luxuriate in the peace. The sun is wrapped in magical, striking colors. Above, the sky is pink, turning to a warm orange and yellow glow surrounding the sun? The clouds are white up high and sinking right down to grey, darkest of blue just above the ocean. The purple just above the horizon starts so soft near the sun and sinks into the black of night. You see the stars beginning to awaken throughout the sky, twinkling to life because the day shifts into the night.

With the darkness settling in, you opt to make your way to your island retreat. The sand feels different now. It is not warm as your feet sink into the calm. The coolness of the sand is still welcoming. One consistent thing is the song of the ocean. Although it's not a whisper, it sings louder, encouraging you to experience the steady cadence, inhaling and exhaling, as you meander your way to your home far away from home. You see the soft glow of the porch light, but you furthermore may see the shadow of the hammock in the yard. The hammock calls to you; you aren't able to close up the ocean's song just yet.

Nestled between two great palm trees, you climb into the hammock. As you sway, you discover your center of balance, focusing your breathing on the faint song of the ocean. Breathing gently in, you allow your feet to rest. Exhalation, you allow your legs to sink into the sturdy net beneath you. Inhaling, your back and stomach settle, and as you exhale, they sigh into the right position of comfort. Resting your arms comfortably, you allow the breath to continue influencing your relaxation. The frogs and insects start to return alive and sing their songs. They are doing not distract you; your music has become your own reflexive action. Inhaling and exhalation is the natural progression. You do not consider actively doing it, your body will still do that as your muscles stay relaxed and your bones settle.

You peer up through the large palm fronds and see every star in the night sky. The moon may be a tiny sliver as if delivering the spotlight of the night sky to the stars, allowing them to share their beauty with you. You start to draw patterns and shapes between the stars. Do you see the bear, the person together with his bow and arrows, the queen sitting upon her throne, the swan flying gracefully through the night? Tracing the connections between each group, do you just see many lines connecting all the stars? Focus harder; check out each star.

Imagine what proportion of life and potential there's to seeing this same star as you at this very moment. You're no different from the other in the big scheme, yet you're a thousand ways unique. You have such a lot inside you, but you're on top of it all. You control where that thought is stored. If it's troublesome, blow it away in a bubble. If it's pleasant, explore it. Allow your eyes to rest just like the remainder of your body. Allow them to be sleepy and asleep. Give the mind control of your entire body; your mind gives you peace, joy, and rejuvenation. Nourish it; enjoy the song of your mind as you drift into oblivion.

Chapter 10:

The Tranquil Submarine

Y ou feel the breeze on your face, cool as it blows over the surreal blue ocean surrounding you. You are on your way to explore the magical world of the ocean by submarine. Excitement is coursing through your body, holding your muscles stiff. You have arrived at the submarine; you stand in line, waiting to walk the stairs down through the porthole. It is finally your turn. As you descend the stairs, you come into the submersible and feel your nerves ramp up a notch as your surroundings close in. Going from the vast ocean openness around you down into a small vessel makes your body feel even tenser. You see the many windows lining the craft, with comfortable seating in front of each.

You eagerly make your way to your seat and sit down, allowing the plush comfort to cradle your body. Your body feels fidgety and antsy as you try to sink into the comfort, try to calm your nerves before this journey. Inhale deeply, allowing the oxygen to reach every organ in your body. Slowly exhale, relaxing the organs as they patiently await the next inhale. As people settle in around you, ignore them, focus only on yourself. Focus on this remarkable journey you're about to experience, seeing a new side of this precious gift of life from below the water's surface. Breathe in, allowing the cool breeze of your breath to travel through your body, down to toes and in between, caressing your feet, allowing them to relax as the breath warms and travels back, ready to be exhaled. Inhale again, this time focusing on the breath to travel down to your hands, in between your fingers, caressing your palms, as the breath warms and travels back to be exhaled. Inhale deeply, allowing the breath to settle your stomach, warming as it caresses your lungs, travels between your shoulder blades and back to exhale. Inhale deeply once more as the breath caresses your brain, warms it, comforts it, and then back to exhale.

You feel calm and relaxed as the pilot's voice comes through the speaker to prepare you for the descent. He tells you to pay close attention to the right side of the vessel as the submarine descends. You turn and see a family of sea lions. A slight shift in pressure reminds you that your body is snug inside this vessel, but let it be a snugness of comfort. The friendly and curious beings approach the vessel, delighting in the bubbles as you descend. Count to see how many sea lions there are. One, two, three, four, five, six, seven; there are seven playful sea lions. They swim quickly around the submarine. One swims up to your window, looking at you as you look at it. Its curious deep brown eyes filled with wonder and excitement, reflecting the wonder in your own. As the submarine continues to descend, the creatures lose interest and swim back to where they were.

Staring out into the vast blueness of the ocean, you reflect on how hectic your life has become. How simple these creatures have it, they just exist and go through every day seeing the beauty in the world, living in it, enjoying it. You start to see small schools of fish, the pilot informs you of some of the species, but you drown out his talking and let it become a soft, lulling murmur in the background. You see fish that are bright blue with yellow tails. They dart this way and that, minding their own business as the vessel passes them by. You see silverfish, some with stripes, some streamlined for speed, some with large graceful fins and a touch of color, traveling in the safety of numbers. All your thoughts from the day are clustered in packs like the fish in this ocean. A small shark soars by, some scatter away, some stick together and ignore the danger. Let's put those thoughts away; just let it be you here, nothing to distract your mind. Visualize the thoughts; now wrap them in a bubble and send them to the surface. They will be there waiting for you on the surface when you're ready for them. Each and every thought should be sent away in a bubble. Watch the bubbles drift to the surface as you keep descending. Let them move further away from you, from your mind, until your mind is clear.

The pilot announces that we are off the coast of an island with lots of unusual creatures; you look closely out your window and see a lizard swim by. Unusual indeed. The pilot tells you that these are marine iguanas, and they are only in this area of the world. The small monster with deep green skin, with hints of red and orange, is beautiful as it swims down onto the vivid green moss-covered rocks. You see a few more as you travel along—some resting on the colorful rocks, some chasing food, some swimming peacefully. The water is so clear and exquisite; it's like being in the world's largest aquarium from the inside. Seeing these creatures in their natural environment, seeing the wonder of their magnificent world is awe-inspiring. You pass through a school of slender fish. It seems there is more fish than water at this point. The fish are so thick the submarine gets briefly dark; it's just thousands and thousands of the narrow-bodied fish outside the windows. Through the thickness, you see a bird glide through the water to snatch some of the fish for an easy meal. It is a penguin. Here in this tropical water, you see a penguin. You listen back in for the pilot to explain that these penguins are also indigenous to these islands. Who would have thought of all these wonderful creatures existing in this one magical place? You see another penguin dive down, do a spin, then dart back up. Its body streamlined for this job of hunting these particular fish.

You realize your body has become tense again as you've moved closer and closer to the window, afraid you will miss something. Sit back, relax, focus on your breathing, and just enjoy what you can see. You will not miss anything. Out your window, you can see a stingray, almost black in color with white dots all over. The stingray gently lifts its wings revealing its white underside as it glides away from the vessel. As you move deeper away from the bright corals and rock and fish, you notice the ocean is more open, cold, and dark. You take the blanket off your chair and pull it snug around you. Blocking out the cold but welcoming the dark as the low lights on the submarine flick on. The fish are more solitary now, hesitant of the vessel instead of curious. You see a large shark pass by, ignoring the submarine... the shark drifts by, going about its daily life. There will be no more descending, the pilot announces, and you're grateful. You feel deep in the ocean, but the peace and quiet you're experiencing is unlike any other.

Out your window, you see a sunken ship. It looks old, lonely, and desolate. But it is now also a haven for many fish away from the coral. You see smaller fish darting around the ship—the local life taking over what was once a part of your world. There is an odd sensation of peace, knowing that you are in their territory, these sharks, these fish, this deep, desolate ocean. This is their home, you are only here to visit, and they don't seem to mind. Some notice you, some don't even bother. They just let you admire. Admire how something old, tired, and broken can become something new and beautiful. This shipwreck is beautiful, harboring so much life around it. The lights illuminate how this ship belongs here now. These animals rely on its existence. This mistake that caused this ship to sink was crucial to the survival of these animals here now. Everything is connected; everything happens for some reason.

You may not always understand, but all you can do is relax and control how you feel, how your mind handles the things around you. You can have a peaceful and meaningful existence like this ship or like the animals around it. You have a purpose, and you will reach that purpose because that is life. The submarine travels on, leaving the ship behind.

As you leave everything behind, your mind feels tired, the coldness of the ocean tries to sink through the walls of the vessel, but the cold doesn't touch you; the blanket is a warm comfort around you. You lie your head back and see through the top glass of the submarine. As your neck relaxes, like the rest of your body, you breathe slowly as a huge sea turtle gracefully glides over the submarine. You can barely see the surface anymore, the dappled sunlight dancing faintly in the dark blue water—the turtle, a dark silhouette, the occasional fish, big and small swimming above. Your body feels heavy but relaxed. Your mind wanders slowly and peacefully as you take in the surroundings of the deep, vast ocean. Close your eyes as you memorize the surroundings to hold with you forever. You will always recall this peace during times of stress; you will be able to close your eyes and see the ocean's surface way above you as the creatures drift peacefully overhead.

Chapter 11:

Visit the Playground

I magine that you are standing at the entrance of a large park. The park was created many centuries ago; sizeable old oak trees border the door. Their trunk is evidence of a long history. A slightly woody fragrance blows towards you from these ancient trees. You can stroke your hands over the gnarled bark of a tree if you like to feel the furrows in the bark; take in the smell of this old tree completely. Take a close look at the crown of the tree and its branches. How expansive and powerful it is, nevertheless the leaves shine juicy green in warm sunlight. Everything around you is pleasant and sunny. The air is pure and bright, charming and refreshing at the same time.

Now go a few steps further and cross the entrance. A large arbor made of green pastures leads you to a square with a large fountain—the square is lined with a green hedge. The fountain is laid out in the middle of the square with many different figures. As you get closer, you can see various fish figures splashing water at each other, gold-colored ornaments of the fountain shine towards you in the sun. You can hear the quiet rippling of the fountain and the gentle blowing of a spring wind, pure, bright, and refreshing.

The path now leads you to a large meadow, which is provided with many flower beds on edge. The flower beds are playfully arranged at different heights. You can see the most mixed spring flowers, small blue flowers, large orange flowers with hanging flower heads, and purple ones. Flower carpets in between there are small stone figures, ornamental stones, which are also partly covered with a carpet of flowers. It smells wonderfully fresh and flowery. Little birds fly chirping across the meadow and peck happily in the field. Other flocks of birds fly over their circles in the park. A bright, fresh wind blows towards you and envelops you with a beautiful floral scent. The sun shines warmly on you; everything is warm and pleasant, calm and clear.

Your further path leads you to an old palace complex. A small summer palace was built many centuries ago in this park with many walkways, small fountains, shrubs, and a wide variety of trees, and everything has now come to life in spring. The trees form their first buds. One of the other trees already shines in a delicate white-pink, the other in an intense bright yellow, and around the tree trunks, you can see small carpets of flowers. They surround the trees and in their bright colors. You feel that it is spring awakening now. The trees and the flowers shine in their blossoms.

On one side of the pleasure palace, you can see a large water surface; with many small hidden benches. You take a seat to enjoy the upcoming spectacle in peace. Your desk is decorated with many ornaments and pleasantly warm. Feel your weight on the seat and the pleasant warmth. Your surroundings smell of fresh, clear water, and an apparent wind gently blows over your shoulders. It is almost like a caress, very gentle and tender, loving; here, you can feel completely comfortable. Everything is calm and pleasant. Breathe in this pure and clear air, and take it in entirely in you in to refresh yourself.

There are many stone figures on the edge of the water surface. A large funnel-shaped stone sculpture stands in the middle of the water. The statistics on the side represent lions, peacocks, eagles, angel figures; from a distance, you can perceive a continually approaching soft noise. A gentle and calm music sound fills the whole environment, and the gentle harmonic sounds envelop everything. Water from the funnel-shaped stone sculpture in the water is now spraying in all directions, from the other figures. Water is also spraying into the middle of the pond—everything tailored to The beat of the music. The water harmoniously adapts to the tones of the melody. It ripples and clinks and weaves around every person who listens, in perfect connection with this place, a place of calm and harmony.

As the melody fades away, the water also pulls back. You continue to look at the park and its vast meadows with many fruit trees decorating your path. Apple trees are already littered with many fragrant flowers, cherry trees stand in full bloom.

The scent of flowers fills your path. Little squirrels jump from branch to branch and climb along with the trees. A sizeable flowering willow lines your way. Their branches hang many meters from the crown to the ground. A whole flock of birds has settled in this Pasture. They now use spring to build their nests. They chirp, argue, compete for the most beautiful bride, fly their races in large arches around the tree, and happily chirp on theirs again Pasture.

Now you are at the last of the park. A long green arcade with small pink flowers leads you past an old greenhouse, which with its old glass windows reflects a calm and reliable permanence. A little playful rock garden is around the greenhouse, small ones. Ducks are chattering in the field and looking for a suitable place for your nests.

You are now back at the entrance and take in the feeling of spring on your journey home. The pure and clear air, the scent of the blossoming trees and plants, the awakening of nature, the happy chatter of the ducks. Happy after their nesting site looking for the feeling of togetherness.

Chapter 12:

Summer Stroll

T he warmth hits my face as I venture out the check the weather, 80 degrees. It's not the longest walk, but rather it certain as damnation isn't the briefest, all things considered. This mid-July dampness doesn't help cause the distance feel any shorter. Two or three stages from the structure, and I have effectively begun to perspire, an achievement I felt I'd reach at any rate 5 minutes in. I can feel it on my temple and at the scruff of my neck, not dribbling but rather barely enough that in the event that I was with individuals, it would make me hesitant. I tie my hair up and trust this walk will merit staying away from the vehicle ride with my sister. I can't resist the urge to feel a twinge of disappointment with the prospect of the cool air from the air conditioner that might have been hitting my face directly at this point.

In spite of the fact that it would have been a short drive, it would have felt like triple the distance with my sister. Just to show up home before this lunch begins, compelling me to collaborate like I completely appreciate the organization of my family and their visitor. I can feel my nervousness rising at simply the prospect of making casual banter with my mother's companions. God forbid I go higher up to pause and rest without my sister or mom remarking on how discourteous I'm being. In some cases, I luck out, and my father allows me to sneak off for a piece, and when asked about my whereabouts, he just states I was sent on an errand. Whenever allowed to miss this, trust me, I seize it. I calculated this walk would give me some peace prior to hurling myself to these social wolves. An idea that happened when attempting to choose whether I should simply leave the store after a warmed contention with my sister. Just as the reality, I'd be advised to shower and change to be "satisfactory," as my mom would say. Peace. That is all I required.

I'm just about ten minutes in, and I've begun to see a decrease in moistness.

Happy to see mother earth is my ally.

As I continue to walk, the climate change begins to feel more extreme, enough to make me set my hair back down. I loosen the sweater I had around my midsection and toss it on, which makes me happy I wore pants. But on the other hand, I wish it hadn't been my most torn loose pair. I can feel a breeze hitting both my kneecaps. I can feel the cold on my nose and cheeks; almost certainly, they'll be red like my face when I make a weak joke at these snacks.

Now I'm part of the way through my stroll with my hoodie up and arms crossed, wanting to keep warm. I begin to see that with the wind came snow. It is anything but light snow;

however, it's insufficient to keep me from completing my stroll; actually, it appears to be more tranquil.

Not an incredible sign for the earth.

Not ideal climate for a mid-July day but rather certainly what I required for this walk. I ought to presumably consider how odd this is and what this could mean. Yet, I don't. There's nothing I could do except for being appreciative of the peace it gives me. It makes the world such a ton calmer. The wind feels like it has frozen a portion of my contemplations. In a short time, I'll hit the more local location, and I'm certain to run into more individuals. I dread this.

I ought to simply sit briefly.

I peer down and look for confirmation that the trees have saved the ground from being over-taken by snow. I sit. I realize I'll be later to this lunch; however, I'm certain they'll be excessively occupied by this unusual drop of snow from mother earth. I can't resist the urge to trust that it'll drop the lunch. I close my eyes, take a full breath and feel exposed. It's not cruel on my skin, more like a reviving inclination. It's an incredible cooldown, not simply from the mugginess that was making me feel like each move I made helped my perspiration organs. Be that as it may, from the contention I had with my sister, a senseless contention. One that came from other profound established issues with her, from an external viewpoint that contention was a joke. I had recently referenced how I wasn't

92

actually anticipating lunch, which she, for some reason, took as an individual affront. She's been assisting our mother with getting sorted out these snacks for quite a long time, each second Saturday of the month. I've been getting lucky and missing for quite a long time while I've been away for school. Yet, presently since I've been home, I've needed to share.

Me hating the lunch was more surface-level; I just couldn't deal with them with my tension. I've had mental episodes formerly and needed to pardon myself. I attempted to leave as serenely as could be expected while realizing I was receiving some menacing glares from my sister.

One year throughout the colder time of year, before I had begun school, I had a mental breakdown during lunch. I was plunking down in the lounge room with a companion of my mother, her better half, and their 19-year-old girl. They had gotten going with some casual chitchat about the climate; it was similar to now. At that point, they proceeded onward to the feared subject, school. It went from where was I applying to? What was I going to study? How were my present school marks? What extracurriculars did I have? Right when I, however, was done, and the besieging of inquiries had finished, they started with talking about how incredible their girl was doing. I was at that point so uncertain of what to do, I didn't have to have somebody to compare myself with. I felt like I was unable to inhale, I began to feel my pulse rise, and regardless of it being so cold out, I felt like I was on fire. I attempted to excuse myself as amenably as conceivable with a stammer or two in the blend.

I was from the vast majority currently setting out toward my room, but my sister made up for the lost time with me. I was through 33% of the route up the steps and met with erupting nostrils. I was so centered around moving endlessly all I truly took from her reproving a few words and some halfway sentences. Disillusionment. Impolite. You don't put effort or make an attempt. Uneasiness. I felt the tears begin to form, and I refused to slowly inhale. As she left, the tear, at last, hit my cheek. I was amazed it didn't make a sizzle. I rather strolled down to the front yard, and I gazed toward the stars as I sunk into the snow.

Very much like I am presently. Very much like then, I let the snow encompass me, and despite the fact that I'm beginning to freeze, it's calm out; my considerations have eased back, and very much like that day, I feel settled once more. Tragically, there aren't any stars out yet. It's shady, and the sun is practically covered up. Increasingly more snow sneaks through parts of the tree, and some snow chips hit my face. I get up and begin making a beeline for the house. When I come to the private, I begin to see youngsters out playing in the snow and concerned guardians attempting to appreciate it with the children. I can hear several grown-ups talking about how it might affect us and the Earth's temperature boost. I can feel my own tension rising a piece, yet I attempt to simply take in the snow. Attempting to prepare myself for whatever will be at my home, however, at any rate, I bought significantly more time as I needed to shower and change. I grin, snow hits my face, and my walk comes to an end as I approach my carport.

Chapter 13:

Autumn Dream

B efore we begin this journey downwards into the deepest realms of our subconscious, let us take a minute to physically, mentally, and spiritually acclimate ourselves into being one with our inner sanctum, our internal workings. We will begin by going to a place of comfort, ideally a bed or a very comfortable reclining chair, and we will relax our bodies to the furthest extent possible. Now, close your eyes, staying firmly on your back, with your arms relaxed at your sides and your legs rested downwards. Take one deep breath in, through your nostrils, counting slowly to four, and one deep breath out, through your nostrils again, counting slowly to four.

Jenny shook her head in dismay as she looked at her child, sitting amid a veritable pile of candy wrappers.

A cold Autumn breeze rolled in through the window, and she got up to shut it.

"What am I going to do with you, kiddo? You are going to be up all night, bouncing off the walls with all that sugar! What was I thinking?"

Kirsty literally bounced on the bed, her gap-toothed grin fueled by entirely too much chocolate and marshmallow.

"Best Halloween ever, Mommy! I got, like, a hundred pounds of candy!"

Jenny laughed. The girl's enthusiasm was, if nothing else, infectious.

"I don't think quite that much, sweetie, but if you did, I'd box most of it up for next year!"

"Ewww!" Kirsty wrinkled her nose. "I don't wanna eat year-old candy!"

"I didn't say you'd have to eat it!" laughed Jenny.

"Maybe we'll give it to your father as punishment for letting you eat so much candy tonight!"

She sighed. Sometimes that man just did not think about things before jumping into them, and Jenny was left cleaning up the mess.

Kirsty giggled uncontrollably. "I bet he'd barf!"

"I'm sure."

"Do you think he would barf so much it'd fill up my candy bag, Mama?"

"Oh, gross, young lady! Let's not talk about such things before bed!"

Jenny reached out and lightly touched the tip of Kirsty's nose with her finger.

"Now, how am I ever going to get you to sleep in this condition? It's an impossible task!"

"What about a story, Mommy?"

Jenny put a finger to her lips and paused in thought.

"You know what? That's not a bad idea!"

She went to the self and picked up a well-worn paperback.

"No, not that one!"

Jenny's fingers glided over to a thin storybook.

"Nope! The big one!"

Jenny picked up the heavy book with the crackling cover.

"Yes!"

As she sat on her daughter's bed, Kirsty managed to bounce even higher in anticipation.

"This book is the best one, Mommy! The stories in it really come to life! Better than the other ones."

"Okay, this one it is, sweetie. Now lay back and let me find a good one."

Though its covers were weathered, as Jenny slowly turned the pages to find the right story, they felt glossy and as new as when she herself was a kid.

"Let me see, let me see...."

One page stood out—a corridor of trees with leaves of red and gold arcing over a long road.

A lone branch had fallen in the road, a slender arm with a single thin shoot reaching away from the main branch.

It resembled a numeral "6," surrounded by falling leaves. As the mother and daughter watched, a few more leaves fluttered lightly to the ground.

"This is perfect for a brisk Autumn night. We have got a toasty fire going downstairs. If you listen, you can almost hear its warm crackle...."

* * *

Glimpses of a sunset through the trees sprawled red, orange, and purple across the Autumn sky.

The wind rustled the branches and fanned the leaves like crackling flames of red and gold that arced overhead.

Jaina felt as though she walked through a warm fire on the hearth itself.

The air was fresh but brisk, with the Fall sweeping through and alive with the energy of changing seasons.

She breathed in deeply, and the air smelled of pumpkin patches, spiced apples, tree sap, and the wood fires burning.

This time of year had a special resonance as Summer gave way to Winter and the changes that swept in before the leaves fell.

Nights like tonight were magic—a living dream.

She almost needed no sleep; to walk down the street on such a night was as invigorating as any night's rest.

As Halloween approached, the world came to life with creatures and half-glimpsed spirits rarely seen outside of this time.

The change was upon the world, in the rich scents that wafted through the air of baking pies, of sweet apples upon the trees, of cold drafts from distant lands, and fires upon the hearth.

Smoke drifted from the chimneys as she passed rows of houses. Orange light shone warmly in the windows against the darkening world. The faded blue scarf she kept wrapped around her neck trailed behind her in the breeze.

There was a field at the end of the street that Jaina had loved since she was a child. It was fenced off now, full of tall grass, and the derelict structures she had played with were long gone.

An old rusted tractor. Concrete chunks left from a house demolished long ago. A small hill with an old well.

She had made up so many stories about the lives that unfolded in that place, the staging site for her adventures into distant castles and faraway lands, or lazy summer naps with her friends while the butterflies flitted slowly overhead.

In Autumn, though, with a scarf around her neck and the change of seasons thick in the air, that field would serve as the gateway to many tales. As the butterflies changed through chrysalis, as the land changed during the Autumn, so did her stories go through metamorphosis.

Jaina walked through the gap in the fence, her fingertips trailing over the cold metal links.

A shiver ran through her as she crossed the threshold, but not because of the cold metal's touch; because she had stepped across the gateway and into another world.

The grass rose up around her steps, rippling in a sudden wind. Lights like fireflies appeared above trails that formed in the grass as hidden things scurried away.

A breath of wind spiraled around her, carrying with it leaves and memory: nutmeg and spice, a steaming hot cup of cocoa in the hands, smoke from the hearth fires, a soft but warm glow as the family huddled around the fireplace and shared stories—the perfect time of year.

Everything was transforming around her. Flowers opened in the field and then fell into slumber again.

Jaina knelt down, hearing a strange sort of symphony in the growth and decline of the flowers.

A hum, like an old playground song, or the music her mother would play as they all danced between kitchen and living room, preparing a celebratory feast as fiery-colored leaves carpeted the yard. And there!

Jaina turned and saw an aged barrel sitting there in the grass amid a cloud of fireflies and butterflies. Water sloshed in the barrel, and the smell of fresh apples filled the air.

The sound of laughter and children's voices followed, and then she saw them, as though they had just sprung from the tall grass.

One of the children was her. Some of them stood on stepstools made of logs. The older ones were tall enough to stand.

They took their turns bobbing for the apples, splashing each other with cold water, giggling like mad.

Leaves of yellow and red swirled about the outside of the scene, like a shifting wall between dream and waking worlds.

Jaina smiled, seeing her older sister push her head into the water before she was ready.

Young Jaina came up sputtering, a leaf sticking in her matted hair. She had been so furious with Melanie that day!

Looking back at it, she laughed. What she would give to go back to that time when her biggest worry was her siblings tormenting her!

Turning to her right, Jaina saw another wall of leaves before her, which parted as she approached.

This time she stepped into a scene she remembered all too well: the night of her thirteenth birthday party.

Jaina's whole family had gathered in the front room with Grandma Gail; that was the last birthday she would ever spend with her grandma.

The old woman smiled at her over her glasses, saving the best present for last. Jaina remembered it well: the very scarf she wore around her neck.

Grandma had knitted it herself over weeks, in Jaina's favorite color: a cool blue, like the Springtime morning sky.

She touched the fabric with her fingertips, still as soft as ever. Some of the colors had faded over ten years, but none of its comfort or warmth.

Grandma Gail had made it especially for those cooler Autumn nights that Jaina loved to explore.

Gail looked up and met Jaina's gaze with her kindly smile. Jaina's heart leaped. A breath caught in her throat.

She stood transfixed as Grandma Gail raised a hand and waved to her.

Of all sitting in the living room, only young Jaina noticed, and she turned her head, searching for whatever her dear grandmother saw.

Young Jaina shrugged and turned back to her scarf, holding it up in the firelight. She wrapped it around her neck and beamed a smile as Gail turned back to her.

Both of their eyes lit up as they shared a special moment that would make one of Jaina's favorite memories.

The leaves shifted again, and Jaina found herself walking beside a creek in a forest. Late afternoon sunlight shone through a golden-red canopy.

She remembered the area well: she had walked here often as a child and later would bring the young man who would one day become her husband on their first tentative date.

This time she was walking behind herself, as a young Jaina balanced precariously walking along a log fallen across the creek.

Older Jaina smiled, knowing what was about to happen. "Watch your step!" she called, and it seemed like her younger counterpart heard something through the mists of dream and memory.

She paused, but it was too late. Her foot slipped on moss, and she tumbled into the creek with a splash.

The water was bitter cold. Jaina came up spluttering and gasping for air, shocked by the frigid water. She laughed and clambered out onto the shore.

Of course, she had to go back to dry off next to a fire in the backyard, but first, she saw what had caused her to slip: a small cocoon hanging on the knot where she was about to put her foot.

She had noticed it at the last second, and trying to avoid it, was thrown off her balance.

Young Jaina found that the timing was more blessed than cursed; however, the chrysalis was beginning to hatch.

A butterfly with drooping wings slowly crawled its way out of the cocoon, taking its first tentative steps as a young adult into an unsure world.

Jaina brushed dripping wet locks of hair from her eyes as she watched, shivering but fascinated.

The butterfly's wings slowly spread as it dried in the brisk Autumn air, patterned blue upon white, trimmed with black. A first few uncertain flaps tested the air.

Both Jainas watched with a bittersweet smile; both faced similar uncertainties, her younger self rapidly growing to meet the greater challenges of the world, and her older self having struggled with those challenges.

Even now, she had to work hard and fight to make her own place in the world.

Yet here, in the dreams of Autumn, those burdens were laid aside. For like the butterfly, as it spread its wings with vigor and took to the sky, she had undergone her own metamorphosis.

From a girl to a young woman who had made her family proud, Jaina had learned to fly on her own as well.

She watched the butterfly as it fluttered up and around her, rising into the shafts of sunlight filtering down through the leaves. A trail of sparkling dust floated behind it like a river of tiny stars.

Jaina reached up and passed her hand through it, and when she drew it back, it seemed like she held for a moment a glimpse of the entire universe shining. Growth. Transition. Metamorphosis.

As the butterfly had undergone its many challenges to become who it was meant to be, so was she undergoing her own changes.

Smiling, the older Jaina turned away. She remembered falling into the creek but until now had forgotten what made her slip.

Now she felt that it was worth the cold and the discomfort to witness something so beautiful.

Her own thoughts rose with the wind like a fluttering leaf, whispering through the trees and into a starry evening sky.

Below her, the forest unfolded like a vast meadow of apple-red and sunshine-gold.

Ribbons wound through it in the form of the streams and creeks, helping to shape a vast tapestry.

The leaves would fall and carpet the ground in royal beauty, and the trees would stand naked in their beauty for a season.

Seeds slept in the earth's firm embrace; buds dreamed upon the branches. A blanket of frost covered all, turning to glisten dew in the morning sun.

Through it, all the land and all its dreaming creatures continued to grow and transform to find their Spring. For now, in Autumn's sweet embrace, the world slept, and Jaina floated above it in peaceful memory.

Chapter 14:
Friday Night Dinner

He really likes chicken. So as today is Friday, I will make roast chicken tonight.

I carefully take the herbs from the cupboard: rosemary, thyme, and bay. I ensure that the vegetables are chopped to match each other in size precisely. Carrot, onion, sprouts, and tiny broccoli florets. I break the garlic into cloves, rubbing butter into the plump pink skin of the chicken with my hands. The vegetables sit happily around the sides glistening in oil. I crack black pepper and salt over the chicken watching the flakes fall over the curved shape. I squeeze lemon juice carefully over it all before placing the lemon inside the chicken. I halve the potatoes and boil them until just soft before throwing them in a pan with oil and fat. The potatoes and vegetables join the chicken in the oven for the final 45 minutes. Right on time.

He will take the 16:54 train from London Waterloo. He will sit in the first carriage of the train tapping away at his phone, too distracted to notice the heat of the rush hour bodies all packed in together. The train takes 28 minutes until he will reach the local village station. He will get off and probably walk to the house because it's a clear spring day. Perhaps he will stop at the corner shop and buy two bottles of Peroni, water droplets dripping down their necks. People will stop him and chat because he loves to talk. At the end of our street, he will pause to check his breath, taking that gold ring from his pocket to slip onto the fourth finger. He will put his phone away and plaster on a smile for me.

He will arrive at 17:45, like always. The grandfather clock in the quiet hallway chimes five times; everything is right on time.

I take a sip of wine; the bitter taste lingers in my mouth for slightly too long. I lean against the countertop, my hand resting on the cool marble. I gaze around the silent kitchen. We had spent months arguing over this kitchen. It was a hot summer two years ago, roaming in and out of various warehouses discussing with designers the color of the marble, the cupboard handles, the fridge brand, the freezer compartments, even the number of toaster slots. For someone who would barely set foot in this kitchen, he had opinions on every square inch of this room. He has opinions on everything. I walk over to the sink and turn the tap to the left, running my hands under the water, perfectly warm. I dry them with one of the soft hand towels hanging next to the sink. I can't help but run my palm over the cool marble, brushing a crumb into the sink. It is a beautiful kitchen.

The house is otherwise silent; the timer, in the shape of an overweight chicken, ticks incessantly from its perch on top of the oven. A bird sings cautiously in the garden, breaking the otherwise perfect peace. I could switch the television on for half an hour to pass the time, the five o'clock news will fill the kitchen with background noise. I can numb myself with the world out there. Or I could catch the end of one of those American afternoon movies on Channel Five. Each one is different and yet exactly the same. Perhaps I could make a dessert, a trifle, or cheesecake. Something he likes. Something that will make him stay.

I know that he likes chicken. Yesterday I made chicken alfredo pasta, the day before a chicken korma, the day before that chicken burgers. The local butcher knows me by face now. That strange lady always coming to buy chicken. I know that he likes chicken, so I make chicken. My days are fairly militant at this point—half an hour of reading after breakfast, walk to the village shops for fresh meat and vegetables, resist the judgment of the local gossip. Of course, I see their faces when I go through the main streets. I watch the faces flash from distaste to faux concern when they catch my gaze. I can imagine the discussions that occur as I pass by out of earshot. 'What did she expect marrying him?' 'Shame such a pretty young woman!' 'Well, if you ask me, she asked for it....'

Strawberries. We have strawberries somewhere in the fridge. I take them out and wash them carefully under the cold tap. I can make some fresh whipped cream to go on top. I know that he likes strawberries. We served them at our wedding. It had been an early summer day, almost the end of strawberry season. There was strawberry juice splashed on several expensive dresses and suits, cream smeared on the dancefloor. There is a picture of that day on a table in the hallway, a place that no one ever pauses to look at. I'm looking up at him adoringly, the intricate lace of the dress following the curve of my back. He is looking straight at the camera, handsome as usual, in some intense conversation with the photographer. An arm loosely thrown around my shoulders distracted as always.

I gently pluck the tiny green hats off the strawberries, throwing away those that are showing early signs of age or softness. I whip the cream by hand, my arm aching slightly from the effort. 17:20. I should set the table. There is a chill in the air in the dining room. I open the doors to the garden, the hairs on my arms raising at the temperature change. I take a fresh tablecloth out of the dresser that his mother handed down to us. She had explained to me how to take care of the wood with painstakingly particular attention as if I were a toddler. I spread the tablecloth wide, lowering it gently to touch the table. I smooth the creases out with my palms. I take two candlesticks out of the cupboard and place them exactly in place before choosing his favorite plates. They are a brilliant white with edges dipped in royal blue. The cutlery joins them on either side, exactly right, just as he likes it.

17:25.

I go up to the ensuite bathroom that adjoins our master bedroom. The stairs creak in the same places. I dab the perfume that he bought me for Christmas on each wrist before touching it softly to my neck. The scent is too sweet, too much vanilla for me, but he likes it. I choose to put on the slinky red dress with a tie waist that he complimented last year at his sister's birthday. I roll barely sheer tights carefully up my legs. I slide my feet into a pair of shoes, buffing slightly at some dirt on the left heel. I look at myself in the mirror. The same sad face stares back; my eyes are dull and dark. I dot concealer around the shadows, covering the traces of the tears. I dab a little touch of lipstick onto my lips, he doesn't like it when I leave a mark, so I blot it several times to make sure it won't.

Downstairs the roasting chicken is filling the peaceful air with glorious scent. The bird is still chirping outside, now with company. Even the birds have company whilst I wander around this empty house. I open the oven and mix the potatoes, turning them over so that they will brown evenly in these last minutes. I take the butter out so that it can come to room temperature. I slice open some bread rolls and pile them together in the basket, placing them off-center on the table. I put down a mat that will hold the hot dish for the chicken. The table is set.

I take a bottle of white out of the fridge. The same one I have already been drinking. Maybe tonight he will want beer instead of wine; I put both glasses on the counter in case. Perfect.

Everything is exactly how it should be. 17:35. He should be off the train by now. I close the doors to the garden so that the dining room can warm up a little. The fresh air has filled the space with optimism.

We could watch a film afterward. Maybe he will want to talk about work. Maybe he will be tired after the office. It has been a long week for both of us. They don't see how he is at home, these women that talk about us behind my back. They don't know how he looks at me, making me feel as though I am the only woman in the world. They don't know how well he loves me. All they know is the stories, the rumors that have continued to circulate. They don't see how he rests his hand on my leg when we watch a film, how he pulls out the chair for me to sit down before him. How safe he feels. The overweight chicken timer is still ticking away. 17:40. Any minute now, he will be here, finally.

The phone buzzes on the counter against the marble. If I ignore it, it isn't real just yet. For this moment, I can be the perfect wife, waiting for her perfect husband to come home and eat a perfect meal together on a Friday night in their perfect house. I know that he really likes chicken. The lump in my chest rises, filling my throat. I swallow my nerves.

The overweight chicken is finally ready, relief against the unbearable silence. I take two oven gloves from the drawer to the right of the oven. I open the oven and let the heat brush my face. I take the chicken out; the skin is perfectly golden and glistening in the light. The smell fills the kitchen, and I forget for a second, a meal this good is just unmissable.

As I slide the chicken over the marble, the phone vibrates again. I glance over at the screen, and my heart tightens; like always, time stops.

'Tried to call, it didn't go through. I'll be late tonight; I'll just stay at the same place; it's easier. Be back tomorrow probably."

Conclusion:

T hank you for making it through to the end of Bedtime Stories for Adults. Let's hope it was informative and able to provide you with all of the tools you need to help you sleep well.

This may be the end of this book, but your odyssey into the depths of your imagination is far from over. I encourage you to reread these stories, becoming more and more familiar with their characters and detailed settings.

You are probably familiar with what it's like to reread books or stories and noticing new things when you revisit them. There are simply things you won't notice the first time around.

The joy of reading can be even greater when you come back to stories you have already read because you aren't only reading to get the story from it anymore. You are reading for the rich detail in the sentences and for a new perspective of the plot and characters since you already know what happens.

Think back to a time when you got really into a book because you so badly wanted to read the next part of the story. These kinds of books do exceptionally well in the market because they make people always want more. While these kinds of books certainly have their own worth, there is one big problem with them, at least if you are trying to fall asleep.

Since you are reading them as fast as possible just to get the story, you don't get to enjoy the smaller moments that make up the character's journey. All you are doing is reading for information, much like you would a textbook. I'm not denying it can be fun, but it is certainly no way to calm down before bed.

Take the most recent book you have done this with. Ask yourself: did you find that it helped you fall asleep when you read it before bed, or did it just keep you up late because you really wanted to know what happened?

Now, it's actually likely that it helped you get to bed to some extent. That's because stories wrap us up in their own world, so you still let go of yourself and your own stresses for a while when you are reading them, even if you are skipping the smaller details to get to what happens next.

However, it is better to read a book of short stories written explicitly to get you to fall asleep. Since you are at the end and you have already enjoyed them, you already know that these stories are still entertaining. They still get your head into its imaginative space and into a world created by words.

But you also know after reading that they were not written for you to simply find out what happens next. Their pacing is nice and steady, so you can enjoy the journey through the story instead of rushing through it to get there as soon as possible.

Therefore, the merit of these stories isn't lost when you read them again. You aren't only reading them to see what happens. You want your mind to create an image given to you by each sentence so you can get your brain to create that image instead of occupying itself with whatever stressful thoughts that will usually keep you up at night. They get you to stay focused on the path you take to get to the end of the story.

The more you became a part of the worlds we sculpted, the easier time you will have letting go of the real world and drifting off to the world of dreams. You can wear the clothes the characters in these stories are wearing instead of wearing your own.

Looking at storytelling from a broader perspective, what the written words are meant to do is give you a new perspective of the world.

The world you perceive can be the world of dreams and people who live very far away from you. It can transport you from the day-to-day drudgery and toil and replace it with a great story.

The truth is, you can't actually turn it off; you can only disengage it by engaging a different neutral network, the default mode network. The best way to engage that network is by reading stories.

Getting your brain engaged in a fictional story can be good for your stress reduction in general. Short stories serve a variety of purposes, and getting to bed is just one of them. You are certain to discover these uses as you continue to read and reread these stories.

CPSIA information can be obtained
at www.ICGtesting.com
Printed in the USA
BVHW040850070621
608930BV00014B/307